Care for the Caregiver

Out
of
Love

A Daughter's Journey
with Her Mom
to the End

Care for the Caregiver

Out
of
Love

A Daughter's Journey
with Her Mom
to the End

Lynn Abaté-Johnson

Table of Contents

"Dear daughter: Be loud, take up space—your voice matters."

–Angela Anagnost-Repke

Dedication

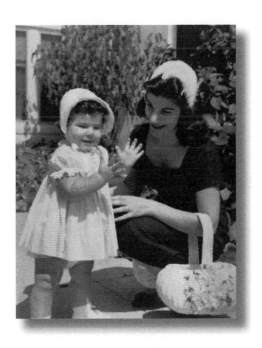

This book is dedicated to my mom, Rosemary Ann Hakim (a.k.a. RAH or RahRah), who has always been my inspiration to thrive, not merely survive.

Author's Note

HINDSIGHT: BE ENCOURAGED.

It has occurred to me while writing this book that I am "writing from the scar, not the wound," as author Glennon Doyle says. I feel fortunate to be in this exact position here and now. My mom took her final breath on May 1, 2017. Recently, I was going through a box of memorabilia and came across many cards, mostly birthday and thank-you cards, written by my mom to me. I think in the first few years after my mom died, this "walk down memory lane" might have triggered some tears in my ongoing grief journey. Most of the time these days, however, memories of my mom bring smiles and sometimes a chuckle. There are poignant and painful moments that hit when I least expect them, as is the process of grief. There's no formula. There are no rules. What I know for sure, and what you may have already experienced, is that on some days you'll carry grief lightly, and on other days it will drop you to your knees. Be encouraged that you are not alone in this journey, although each is uniquely ours.

I didn't have a "touchy-feely" relationship with my mom; however, I feel happy and at peace with the relationship we had. It wasn't all roses, and in fact, at times, it was two headstrong women who were "raising" each other. I was her firstborn. She was my biggest cheerleader as well as my harshest critic.

One of the toughest and sweetest lessons I learned during my final years with my mom is this: Live your life now in such a way that you mitigate regret in your own life to the extent you are able. It's one of the healthiest ways to process grief, both before and after the death of a loved one. No regrets. This became my mantra through those "cancer years."

This book was originally going to be about my mom and her experience through ovarian cancer. What it has become is my very personal and transformational journey—one guided with love from my mom and so many others—as you'll see in the pages to follow.

My mom's note to me toward the end of her life.

TIMELINE OF MY MOM'S OVARIAN CANCER JOURNEY

February 4, 2011: original diagnosis = stage IIIC ovarian cancer

February 7, 2011: removal of all visible cancer in debulking surgery: complete hysterectomy, removal of peritoneum, omentum, part of colon (resection), abdominal lymph nodes, appendix

April 2011: began chemotherapy (aggressive clinical trial)

June 15, 2011: discontinued chemotherapy

March 13, 2015: resumed chemotherapy

December 18, 2015: began oral chemotherapy (Lynparza)

February 2017: resumed chemotherapy (via IV, as the cancer metastasized around lungs, liver, and spleen areas)

April 11, 2017: chemotherapy ended. Entered hospice with the goal of staying comfortable, while taking IV vitamin therapies to allay symptoms (aches and pains mostly in back and stomach with intermittent shortness of breath).

May 1, 2017: final breath in her own bed. No machines and no morphine. All is well. She is at peace and completely FREE of dis-ease.

OVARIAN CANCER OVERVIEW

Don't ignore symptoms of this silent disease!

Too often, ovarian cancer is only caught once it has entered stage IV (80 percent of cases).

Symptoms: Bloating, increased abdominal size, pelvic or abdominal pain, feeling full quickly when eating, an urgent or frequent need to urinate, unusual fatigue

Tests: New tests are evolving fairly frequently. For us, one marker for ovarian cancer was the CA-125. Things change rapidly, so I encourage you to look into organizations like the National Library of Medicine.* Be sure to search online for the most current information for your case.

*Please visit the Resources section at the end of the book where I've included a small sampling of available source materials. Additionally, you can always search online using the keywords relevant to you and your diagnosis.

Introduction

In a moment, my life as I knew it turned upside down.

Wait. What?

Mom, why are you tired during the middle of the day?

Why do you have to lie down?

You never take naps or lie down when the sun is up.

Your stamina is never diminished.

You have endless energy.

You run circles around everyone, including your children.

What's going on?

You can't do your exercises without being winded, and your tummy, feet, and ankles are constantly swollen.

What the heck?

Something is really wrong.

It has to be. Dare I force you to visit a doctor?

I don't want to face any horrible news and neither does anyone else, yet we need to act, and quickly.

Denial is no longer an option . . .

And now we have the answer. It's ovarian cancer, stage IIIC.

I was "this many years" old, well into adulthood, when the pillar of my world, my strong, feisty little mama, received this life-threatening diagnosis.

In these pages, my pledge to you is to help normalize the complete and utter jolt of the disorienting journey that I took with my mom, Rosemary Ann Hakim, a journey you may be on right now with your own loved one. I'm committed to supporting you in your caregiving journey; I am committed to addressing your fears, anxieties, conflict, joy, humor, doubt, rage, sadness, anger, guilt, and more.

They say that hindsight is 20/20, and while I realize it's a cliché, I've noticed it to be true in my life, especially since my mom died. I offer insights about the nitty-gritty in the form of actual journal entries I wrote in the moments of caregiving. Each chapter starts with at least a part of one of my online journal entries from my mom's home, hospital rooms, doctors' offices, emergency departments, and all the places we found ourselves during what I call the "cancer years." Very likely, you'll identify with some of these details in serving someone you love as a caregiver through dis-ease, illness, treatment, death, and grief. Following my journal entries, I share my perspective in the aftermath, years later, relating to how I learned more about myself through those years. Transformation through my grief is one way that I look at it. The bottom line is that I'm with you. There is care for the caregiver in these pages.

Writing the online journal entries helped me disseminate vital information about my mom's condition to our whole community, near and far. It's part of the basis for me writing this book. I wrote nearly every day for most of that first year (2011). The original purpose was to make communication as efficient as possible and to provide a general overview of my mom's daily life. I wrote to pass along basic information, detailed information, and perhaps, at times, too much information (especially when it came to my mom's pooping milestones, for example). I also wrote to reassure faraway loved ones that my mom was being cared for by us and her medical practitioners. And while I was at it, I also wanted to help educate, as that was a big part of our "why." My mom was very committed to having people learn from her experience (and the fact that she eventually tested positive for the BRCA2 genetic mutation). Another aspect of my writing in the online journal back then was inserting some humor into a very scary, ugly, messy, dark circumstance. I figured when we weren't in tears over our prospects and concerned about what the future held, we may as well laugh, smile, and joke around here and there.

You will notice throughout that I write disease in this manner: dis-ease. This is a metaphysical term, as I understand it. It is a manner of describing that our bodies/whole systems are not at "ease" (out of balance) when we are in the throes of an illness. This helps frame the mindset in a more holistic way, which opens more pathways to bring harmony to our systems through whatever modalities we choose.

"Dis-ease is dis-connection. Healing is re-connection."

–Dr. Sarah Campbell, Instagram

Your Life Prepares You for Life

February 6, 2011

We just found out some scary news.

We knew nothing before now.

Our little mama has been diagnosed with stage IIIC advanced ovarian cancer and will be undergoing an aggressive treatment plan led by a brilliant gyneco-logical–oncological surgeon we were referred to. He has been practicing for twenty-two years. Our mom is very confident in his credentials and capabilities.

Needless to say, one of us kids will be camped out 24/7 at the hospital in her room with her. We are cur-rently in production mode, getting a pre- and post-op nutritional protocol going, calendars for who is on duty, and all her tests, doctor information, etc. organ-ized into a binder, including notebooks for note-taking at the hospital.

To say that we are scared is an understatement. Her pain is pretty extreme right now. Her legs, stomach, and feet are incredibly swollen, and when she coughs, it hurts her a lot. We will be sending updates as we go along. She loves cards and photos, and if you can get some snail mail to her, that would be awesome, as it helps lift her up and makes her feel loved and appreciated.

Much love and gratitude from all of us here on Team RahRah.

While in shock, I started an online journal as a way to communicate with family members about the day-to-day moments of my mom's cancer journey. To say we were completely unprepared as a family is an understatement. And yet, there's a paradox at play here. We were completely prepared for the six-and-a-half-year journey, plus the aftermath, ahead of us. How was this possible? Our mom raised us to step up, educate ourselves, be productive, and adapt, all without complaint or falling victim to the circumstances. She taught us to be decisive and to take action, even at the risk of making the wrong choice. She taught us to research, to make informed decisions, and to create systems and structures to ease the burden as much as possible. My mom was one of the most pragmatic people I know to this day. When there was a fight to be had, she rolled up her sleeves and dove in. While she had such a soft, loving heart, especially when it came to children, she was also fiercely independent and ready to support the underdog in almost any situation.

I share my most intimate moments and discoveries here with you, using a fraction of those online journal entries written between 2011 and 2019 (some entries are milestone markers in the years since she died). I've added reflections from my various perspectives, then and now. Some of the inquiries dive into these questions:

What tools did I use to navigate this new journey through to the end of my mom's life?
How did the experience impact and eventually change me?
Who was I when it all started and who have I become?
How did I hold my vision of being a strong, capable, loving daughter rather than a victim of our circumstances?
How did I manage to thrive after losing my longest-standing cheerleader and confidante?
Was it worth it?

Overall, I wouldn't have traded this journey for anything, although even writing these words now, I'm fighting with myself to admit it. I certainly never wanted my mom to have to deal with all those years on the ovarian cancer roller coaster. I certainly don't want her dead. There are so many times I wish she were here. I often envision picking up the phone to check in with her, to tell her something funny or about something I'm celebrating, to share stuff I'm sad and miserable about, and so much more.

As the days of that first year unfolded, I found myself in the role of deer-in-the-headlights. I was flying by the seat of my pants and making my mom's cancer diagnosis all about me. In the beginning, I did a great job of navigating, but I also did a really shitty job. In the end, I know I didn't have control of the ultimate outcome. On the other hand, I like to think that my mom felt loved right through to that morning she departed, in her own bed, very sweetly and quietly. This was indeed a gift for me and for her.

As a loving caregiver, my wish for you is that you fully experience everything that comes up as you awaken to what's new and what's the same with each day you are given with your loved one(s). And I'm committed to having you feel comforted by knowing I'm with you there in spirit, at your service.

Further Inquiry

I kept an online journal as a way of communicating with faraway friends and family at first, and later, something I realize now, as an outlet for my grief. Have you considered keeping a journal? What other ways can you stay connected with people and channel your grief?

"She looked at her old life one more time, took a deep breath and whispered, 'It's time. I'm ready for my new story to begin.'"

–unknown

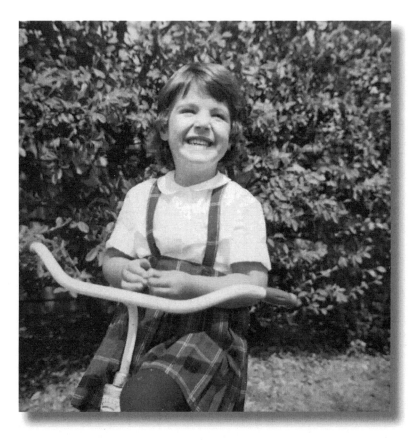

This little girl is learning to thrive without Mama.

Who Is Your "A" Team?

*In true RAH fashion, she is late for surgery. LOL!
She is in high spirits, having a chest X-ray now, and
then an ultrasound on her swollen legs. It's going to
be a long night, and it's only the beginning.*

*RAH is really strong, as you know. Her pre-op
chest X-ray was great. The ultrasound on her swollen
legs ruled out clots (very common with cancer, as it
thickens the blood).*

*We took out her contacts and gave her lots of
kisses. We told her, "DON'T go to THAT light, and
if you have any scary dreams, just replace the images
with your grandchildren giving you lots of hugs and
kisses." We made her laugh a lot during pre-op and
read to her from all your comments. She's in surgery
now, feeling your love, people. Thanks so much.*

*Humorous story from the waiting room. We're
sitting here, so tired that we are finding the weirdest
things to be funny, like the giant fish tank we are*

staring at. My sister Nicole just noticed a huge fish pooping. I said, "It was bound to happen."

No word yet from surgery—which is cool with us because we know this surgeon is meticulous; he's not messing around. He knows what and who is at stake for us, so he's taking his time, confident in his work, cherry-picking each and every spot that needs to be removed. And yet, we are still kind of in shock, in a way, even though we are here, in the hospital, waiting. Nicole says that she feels like we're in a movie.

These were the surreal moments, the ones where we looked at each other once in a while, thinking to ourselves, what the hell is happening here? Is it really my mom in that hospital bed, hooked up and unable to speak (with that "garden hose" down her throat), all bloated and weak, in ICU?

What's going to happen today? Tomorrow? How long is this going to go on?

And for me, personally, I kept wondering whether my mom was going to die imminently. And if so, what was I going to do without her in my life? She couldn't die. She's my mom! I never imagined she'd get cancer and die from it. It seems like every thought I had at that time bounced between *oh-my-gosh-my-mom's-going-to-die!* and *how can I help save her life?*

And so, the journey of discovering how to navigate the dark and surreal unknown became my mission. How did I normalize all that was happening? First, I had to place my focus on what I was able to control while embracing what I could not. I remember thinking of others in my circles of family and friends who I could rely on for my own support as well as my mom's. I started to organize thoughts and make notes and began to create systems and structures that I knew would come into play as we navigated all the "mechanics" of this journey. I also felt all the emotions that arose. A small group of close friends became caregivers for this caregiver. Be sure to seek out those friends—the ones who can swoop you up and take you for a change of scenery or for a quick cuppa or walk in nature. This will help center your spirit, soul, and emotions and give you a place to simply *be*. Ask for the support you need. If it's a challenge for you to do that, as it was for me, I suggest gently practicing it in small ways.

Further Inquiry

Who do you have in your circle that you can count on for support? This may involve stepping out of your comfort zone. The sooner you do it, the better you and the people in your care will be because of it. Write down their names now and be specific about where you think they can help. If this process feels uncomfortable, keep in mind that it is another opportunity for growth.

"If you've been a caretaker for your whole life, receiving care when it shows up will require a major adjust-ment. Adjust. You're worthy of care."

–@DrThema, Twitter

Navigating a New Routine

As the sun rises beautifully, magically, over the local mountain range, we are all envisioning RAH's blood pressure rising just a bit more so she can pass the next round of tests that will enable the ICU professionals to extubate her, and then, a day or two after that, release her to a room. We don't want to rush anything, but you know how we sometimes get an expectation in our heads and then cling to a number (of days in ICU), for example. It's human nature—the report from RAH's overnight nurse is that she rested comfortably without a peep or a cough through the night. She is still putting out a good amount of fluid through the surgical drains. The nurse tried to wean her off the blood pressure meds, but her BP dropped, so he put her dosage back to where it was for now. At least she was comfy (I guess as comfy as could be!).

We have much gratitude for all your encouraging prayers, thoughts, and wishes. I am envisioning taking

RAH out for a walk to soak up some of the sunshine we are blessed with here in Northern California. Very soon.

Letting go of expectations and my timeline was a learning curve, to put it lightly. I was used to being in control, of knowing what to do, of keeping life organized. This new and unwanted routine was a challenge. I was helpless on some days, hoping my presence was enough to comfort my mom while she was picked and prodded at. Normalizing this new timeline took a great deal of trust and surrender.

My mother raised me to see a bigger vision when I'm confronted by a challenge. When I was a little girl, she'd use her words very gently to calm me down and to take a step back. It's funny to notice it and repeat it here. Before this experience, I didn't have this memory of my mom helping me pause, step back, and breathe. And now I'm remembering that she did do that. It was very much in line with what I am learning and practicing today (it's called being Co-Active in my life and business), which is tapping into my "inner leader" to find what is already there . . . the innate "knowing." My mom always knew that I had this skill in me, and it's likely a big reason she would get so frustrated with me as an adult.

So, when she needed me to calmly step up and lead, I was able to muster up that energy I already had inside me to be of service to her and to help guide my family in ways that were uniquely suited to me, including my organizational skills, my decisiveness, and my fierce attention to details in the midst of those shit-hitting-the-fan moments. My mom counted on me for that and more. I was able to step up out of love and out of necessity. For me, it's proven to be a powerful combination. In daily life and when a crisis hits, it translates to being reliable, capable, and incredibly loyal, like my mom was.

My business training and experience has enabled me to break things down into manageable bites. I realized very quickly (because I felt it in my chest and pit of my stomach as soon as I knew something was horribly wrong with my mom's body) that if we didn't organize, strategize, and systematize her cancer journey, we'd be in big trouble and miss so much of the necessary daily details. We were in the dark and we needed to help ourselves see what wasn't visible to us. Thus, our systems of charts, tracking, and checklists made all the difference as we grappled with what was right in front of us at any given time.

This system helped me let go and gave me a sense of security that I was doing everything I could for my mom. In a weird way, the practice of using these systems built up my belief and confidence in our family and community that we would make it through together.

Here is an example of a checklist we used daily, and it was a dynamic list, of course. You are welcome to use it for your own inspiration. Create checklists that work for you or have someone help you with it (remember your team?). It will help, I can assure you of that.

Daily medication: Please CHECK ✓ when done

TODAY'S DATE: _____ **TIME:** _____

EVERY MORNING UPON WAKING

SENNA X 2
THYROID X 1
ZOFRAN X 1 on tongue
"SPECIAL" chocolate section = ½ to 1 dose
("special"/cannabis) Chocolate Chip Cookie (circle one)
FOR PAIN, EITHER (NOT BOTH):
MOTRIN X 2 OR NORCO X 2 (circle one)

NIGHTTIME/BEDTIME

TODAY'S DATE: _____ **TIME:** _____

And so on with the list of current (and ever-changing) medications.

Further Inquiry

What expectations are you carrying around that are out of your control? Creating a system will help you, as well as practicing faith and surrender.

"Empathy is a strange and powerful thing. There is no script. There is no right way or wrong way to do it. It's simply listening, holding space, withholding judgment, emotionally connecting, and communicating that incredibly healing message of 'You're not alone.'"

–Brené Brown, *Daring Greatly*

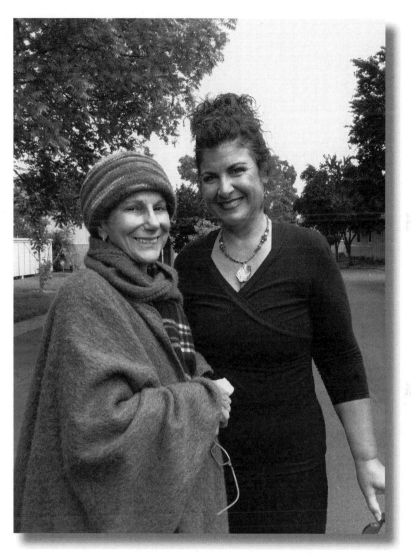

Short chemo walks to keep the strength up.

What To Do When You Don't Like Your Options

Well, folks, we struck the ICU nurse pool jackpot with the evening shift change . . . cha ching! RAH got a new dress (okay, okay, it's a hospital gown), all fresh sheets, and even a back rub with Jojoba oil from the gorgeous and wonderful "K." Plus, we just met his coworker, "E." Both are equally adorable. Sweet and wonderful with my mom. "E" said, "You three look like triplets," because we posted a photo of RAH from pre-surgery days, and he sheepishly said that she looks more like our sister than our mom (no offense taken. We like it when people say that, since we are so secure with our ages . . . ha ha ha). These guys are also extremely competent, we noticed. In fact, other nurses are coming to "K" with questions, and he is a really great multitasker. RAH is resting comfortably after her ordeal of getting her sheets and gown changed. She didn't like it while it was happening, but Nicole

LYNN ABATÉ-JOHNSON

gently talked her through it. It was kind of painful to watch, but it only took six minutes (yes, of course I timed it. You know me and my mom!). They turned her on one side, held on to her, then turned her to the other side and got the job done without too much residual discomfort. Afterward, Nicole rubbed RAH down with oil, moistened her lips, and she is now listening to soothing music on the headphones and is completely relaxed again.

Mostly, we had amazing nurses, doctors, and hospital staff. Once in a while, we did not. I remember clinging to every word that was said by every medical professional, then weighing those words against my own senses. I was keenly aware of the "global" effect and impact that my consciousness brought forth, things like my intuition, my social and intellectual skills, my love for my mom and her care and comfort, and my concern for my siblings, nieces, and nephews, plus all the people who were reading my journal entries and commenting on them every single day.

As the eldest of my mom's five children, and with definite ideas and opinions of my own (read: recovering control freak and overly responsible), I took in as much as I could handle. I did my best with what I had at the time to disseminate information, comfort, reassure, and love to the extent my capacity would allow, moment by moment. I remember being inwardly freaked out when my mom was in ICU after her initial debulking surgery. She was intubated for ten days! Every morning we were told that it was too risky to extubate her and that they would keep trying. Ugh! I knew for a fact (because I could see it in her swollen, intubated face—her eyes were almost swollen shut!) that she wanted *out* of that ICU.

At one point I think Nicole and I knew we needed another opinion, so we went to a senior doctor's office in the hospital to try and "humanize" our mom. We let them know how she was feeling and what she was experiencing. We spoke for her as best we could. We included all the details about how traumatizing it was day after day for her. So, I believe we shifted some energy once we made the choice to have that conversation. And it all wound up okay after all that.

Situations like these were rare, and I have more positive things to say about the hospital staff than anything else, specifically because of the systems I had in place when I was presented with options that I didn't like but had to deal with nonetheless.

My mom was my original example of a community builder (this is my current avocation in my daily life). She was kind and considerate to people from all walks of life. She showed up with curiosity when meeting new people and asked questions she was genuinely interested in. She engaged people, connected different people together, and in her younger days, she loved to have gatherings at home. In her older years, she volunteered for various organizations she was passionate about, and in her retirement years, even throughout the cancer years, she volunteered at her grandchildren's school nearby. She was a true giver. Through her cancer journey, she continually embodied community, love, energy, and transformation day by day, month by month, and year by year, thankfully.

As was my mom, I've been an extrovert and a social butterfly my entire life, so I viewed my interactions with hospital and other medical staff as opportunities to humanize this experience, something that had me scared shitless most of the time. As frightened as I was, I also strove to establish relationships with every shift of medical caregivers, with the intention of having them familiar with my mom. This also seemed to benefit each of the professional teams, because in their increasing familiarity, even as shifts changed, there was more flow and relative ease. There was always a family member present to advocate for my mom, so I felt it was important to get to know the people who were on the front lines alongside us. Something I didn't expect, given that I am keenly aware that the way I tend to show up can be intense and intimidating for some, is that we were embraced. The heightened level at which we were present and paying attention to every detail of my mom's care was welcomed by the staff.

Instead of being insulted, defensive, or offended (which we were braced for, for some reason), the staff were welcoming and grateful, and they went out of their way to remark about how fortunate we were as a family to be able to be in that position of detailed care and support. Since that period in my life, I've learned that our health-care system, while it worked fairly well for us, is severely lacking in terms of many factors, not the least of which is the care for our frontline workers and the complexities of our system being holistic. In other words, I've become very interested in our health-care system becoming a system that supports caregivers and patients in more creative and comprehensive ways. I believe that as the years progress, we have had more caring individuals who are more aware and tapped into resources that are evolving. We have a long way to go, and I will be listening to learn how I can be part of creative solutions in our health-care systems in the future. I saw, and continue to see, so many disconnects in how we approach health care in the United States. We are long overdue for some important paradigm shifts. For example, providing reports—every single type of report—to the patient whose name is at the top of the report, easily, promptly, and automatically, without having to ask. It would also be helpful to automate systems so that medical offices and extended-care offices, including hospital systems, are tied together seamlessly so that no patient care or history details are overlooked in the health-care system. These are basic necessities that seem to be largely missing. Some systems are gradually coming together, but in my recent experience, most are still lacking in terms of seamless communication.

My hope is that we begin to make connections and learn to lean into each other for systems and solutions that work for all people, regardless of the resources patients and their families have available. In our case, I provided every medical office with a fax number and a written request to have all reports faxed automatically to me. It's what my mom demanded, and it's one of the systems we put in place from day one (I have an electronic fax account that makes it easy to receive and organize reports/data that's critical to track, especially in acute scenarios).

Further Inquiry

Have you created any helpful systems or practices in your daily caregiving life? If not, feel free to use anything I have here. Is there anything you would add after reading this chapter that could simplify things further? Write down your ideas so you can come back to them later.

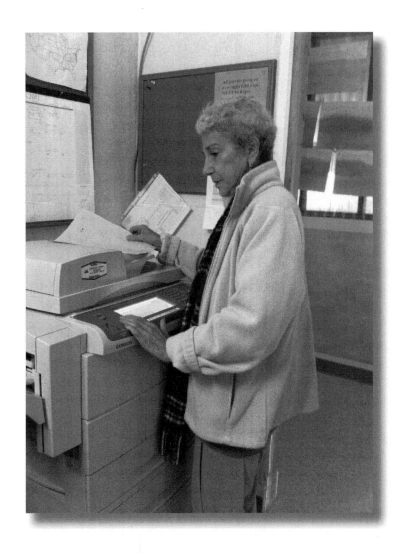

Always volunteering, serving others at her grandchildren's school, out of love.

"There is no controlling life. Try corralling a lightning bolt, containing a tornado. Dam a stream and it will create a new channel. Resist, and the tide will sweep you off your feet. Allow, and grace will carry you to higher ground. The only safety lies in letting it all in—the wild and the weak: fear, fantasies, failures, and successes. When loss rips off the doors of the heart, or sadness veils your vision with despair, practice becomes simply bearing the truth. In the choice to let go of your known way of being, the whole world is revealed to your new eyes."

–Danna Faulds

Too Much and Not Enough

"Land of the Beep and the BRAVE," I remarked to my sister a couple days ago. "If I never hear another one of these machine beeps for the rest of my life, it will still be too soon." But the upshot (there's always an upshot) is that these machines can be magical in all their science and technological foundations. We are continually grateful for the work being done to help RAH get on to the next step. One of her surgeons was in this morning. He remarked positively on all RAH's numbers, signs, and "beeps." He examined her physically, looked at the incision site (54-stitch "zipper" up her trunk—looking great), said she was "a little quiet in her bowels" but that it was nothing to be alarmed about considering there's not much going into her body anyway (in the way of food to be eliminated). The pulmonary doctor was in as well and checked RAH for signs that she is ready to be extubated (we know she would love this!). We introduced him again

to RAH and told him that if he would call her by her name, it would sound a lot like her father speaking to her, which would be comforting for her. (Grandpa's Chaldean/Aramaic accent was beautiful, and this particular specialist had a similar one.)

There was a collective sigh of deep relief for my mom across the country when she was extubated. A dear friend wrote:

Yahoo! So happy to hear the great news! I've been following this journal since you went in for surgery, RAH. You did a great job raising those kids of yours— they have been there at every step and are trying to make the most of each day, whether you know it or not. You better warn the rest of the hospital about what's comin'!

Since I wrote this journal entry, as a "newbie" to the whole cancer and caregiving life, I'd like to think I've become a bit more mature and patient in the realm of advocating assertively (and sometimes aggressively) in the context of collaborating with the medical practitioners charged with my loved one's care. At the time, I didn't want to show these amazing professionals in any sort of dim light in the journal entries; however, I felt the tension between advocating for my mom assertively and aggressively at many moments through the years. It was always a delicate dance, and by that, I do not mean to be "walking on eggshells" or tip-toeing around. That's such a waste of everyone's energy, and it's completely unnecessary. However, there is a certain "finesse" that comes with maturing through the circumstances. My husband, Corey, might call it "reading the room." And there was also my mom's voice in my head, even when she could not say the words while intubated: "Be nice, Lynn." So, this was a struggle and a practice for me all those years (and dare I say still today given my nature to have a direct approach in most things).

In those early days after my mom's big surgery, she was kept in the ICU because they weren't able to remove the "garden hose" from her throat. I can still feel that desperation even as I write these words. Another struggle was the contradiction between what my mom taught me and how I wanted to behave in a given moment. My mom always taught us all to be kind, and she was especially deferential to medical professionals. And so, even when I wanted to challenge or question a circumstance where we were dependent on said professionals to care for her, I zipped my mouth and would sometimes nod in acceptance so as not to appear to be "too much." I did not want to seem overbearing, opinionated, or contradictory. Even though it felt out of alignment for me, I used to let go of what I wanted to express so that my mom felt respected and (literally) obeyed. "Be kind. Be nice." There are new dimensions of these terms that I am only now discovering.

One distinction I'm learning is about being true to myself as well, even in dire circumstances. This helps give me balance, and it's something I can feel in my body.

In a recent conversation with close friends, we talked about the paradox of being seen as "too much" while also having this inner feeling of not being "enough." I'm learning it can be both/and. I'm learning to embrace paradox, which I used to think was contradictory and disingenuous. It is quite the contrary, something I know now especially since my mom died. Both can be true at the same time. My too-much-ness is neither good nor bad. It only has meaning that we, as individuals living in our own skin and our own lives, attach to it. I am actually able to embrace my "much-ness" with love for being exactly who I am and exactly who I am not.

For those who we may be "too much" for, they are not "our people." Yet we can still love each other and wish the best for one another. The whole "enough-ness" issue is something that is all too common, especially in women. It's that saboteur, that inner voice that says all kinds of mean things to us.

My mom's example of being kind to all those who walked into her hospital rooms over the years, as well as those who helped her at home, hits differently now. Even in the time since her death, I'm remembering, unlearning, and learning this lesson . . .

to be kind to myself also. I have come to realize that if I spoke to people with the same meanness with which I speak to myself, I would have no one around me, ever! This is my ongoing leadership journey today.

Thus, in honor of my mom, as uncomfortable as it feels (because I conditioned myself to be hateful toward myself), being kind to myself is a new normal for me, and it's taking practice.

Although the message I hope to convey in sharing my stories here is one of encouragement and love, I realize and acknowledge that during times of extreme fear, worry, crisis, and uncontrollable circumstances, it often seemed impossible to be true to myself.

How do I "fit in" with the new system I've been thrust into?
What do I say when I disagree with a medical professional or question someone else's approach?
How do I navigate all the advice coming at us?
What makes sense for my mom? For me? And what does not make sense?

Telling people to "be yourself" doesn't cut it. As human beings, we are conditioned in one way or another. As years pass, we tend to take on distractions that cause us to forget who we truly are at our essence (hint: our essence is love). It's often said (in some form or another) that as babies, we had no fear, no rational thought, and that all kinds of "conditioning" was laid on us as we grew. Nature/nurture. Conform, get along, be afraid, don't trust yourself or others . . . so much crap!

Normalize that thrash. I consider "thrash" to be my inner dialogue when I have opposing conversations happening in my head. This happened far more often than I thought it would. It took me many years to realize I didn't need to "round out" my edges. There has been plenty of other work going on in honing who I am, as I hold many unique identities. So that's what I've focused on since my mom died: discovering my own identities. How I fit (or do not fit) into the systems I've been a part of. And as a community builder, it's ironic that I also generate and nurture communities in my personal and business life that challenge me while simultaneously leveraging those "edges." Over the years, it becomes more and more stimulating as I continue to learn about myself and how I relate to who I think I am, my communities, and the world as a whole.

I've been supported in all those ways, mostly to become truer to myself, plus more authentic (to coin what has become a buzzword) and more curious.

Today, I have way more questions than I have answers. What a contrast to those younger years when I thought I needed to have it all figured out and know all the answers. I did not. I'm not always in control. I practice relinquishing control more often than not, and it's a lifelong journey of discovery and self-love. Caregivers need to relinquish control, be themselves, and do and be what and who they can in any given moment. Easy? No. Worth it? Yes!

Further Inquiry

What beliefs have you held since you were young that you can now embrace as a force for power in your own life? I find when I ask myself these types of questions, the answers begin to unfold, usually in the form of circumstances where I feel "tested." It's often uncomfortable until I embrace it and go with it—putting my curiosity about myself in the driver's seat rather than my fear or resistance.

"You will always be too much of something for someone: too big, too loud, too soft, too edgy. If you round out your edges, you lose your edge."

–Danielle LaPorte

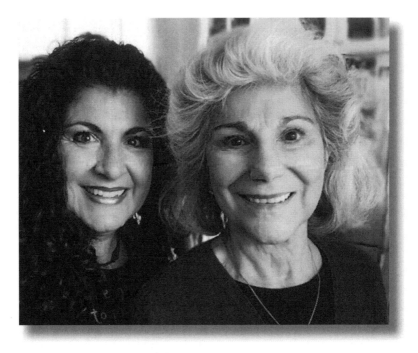

Our holiday pics are precious to me.

*"Don't mistake assertive-
ness for aggression. Being
assertive is advocating
for your interests. Being
aggressive is attacking
other people's interests.
Standing up for your ideals
doesn't make you pushy—
it stops you from being a
pushover. It's not selfish—
it's self-preservation."*

–Adam Grant, Twitter

Community Building

If you ask me today what I predict for my mom, I really see her spark and feel super confident that she will rally and break the cycle of malnutrition at some point. I have no idea how or when. It just feels like she will do it. That's all I've got. She is back to taking charge, asking questions, and writing things down in her notebook, and although she has some issues with clarity at times, she is still as sharp as ever. And, as I have told people all along, she's still my mom . . . still the "boss of me," that's for darn sure!

I walked into her room this morning to find her engaged in a conversation with an X-ray technician about what parts of her body my mom wants to focus on with the X-rays. She said that her chest hurts when she coughs and she wants to check it all out, so they did a full chest X-ray and a couple other slides of her right side where she was complaining of pain. The chronic cough she'd had for twenty-plus years has not been triggered too much, except for when she eats dairy, gluten, and citrus (except lemon). So, this is progress. We just don't want to go backward if we can help it. We need to keep even the tiniest bit of forward momentum. RAH told Nicole tonight that she wants to show 2 lbs of weight gain on the scale tomorrow (we think it's because she's dipped down below 82 lbs again, something she doesn't want us to know, as she was a little cagey when the nurse came by with the scale this morning). We'll see how it goes. We really hope and pray that she'll gain back EVERY pound she needs to have, especially the muscle mass she's lost.

Thank you for being right there with us, cheering us all on, especially RAH. You each make a difference as part of the whole, loving, healthy, and strong community forged with kindness, love, and generosity for our little mama.

Welcome to my mom's large and in-charge presence. She was always comfortable with anyone who was in the room. Whether it was at the hospital, medical offices, her grandchildren's school, her quaint little neighborhood, or the grocery store, my mom could make people feel welcomed, engaged, and at ease. In the small community she adopted in Northern California (after her retirement in Michigan), we loved introducing her to our friends, all of whom became quickly enthralled with her. Consequently, out of her years of service in our tight-knit community, when we needed help caring for her (to the extent she was comfortable and organized enough), people raised their hands and showed up in many ways, large and small. And those people still remember her and tell stories about their encounters with the legendary and beloved RahRah when I run into them in passing in the town where my mom lived and died. My grief process has been lifted in endless positive ways because of my mom's passion for community building.

As much as she was the original community builder, she was a brilliant marketer as well. And this was before these terms were popular. In many ways, my mom's passions were hardwired in me right from the start of my life. She was a foodie. I'm a foodie. She was a marketer. I'm a marketer. She was a community builder. I'm a community builder. In short, my mom was seen as a "maven" in these areas and many more, over her lifetime, and in her various communities.

There was a time when I hadn't put all this together. This awareness really began to unfold during those cancer years, and since her dying breath, it's become more and more clear that my mom is with me at a cellular level. I think we often resist or shirk information that appears right in front of us until we are ready to receive certain messages, or "wisdom" if you will.

Where I may have fought the similarities I had with my mom in my younger years, I learned to embrace the dark and the light sides present in both of us. It's such a liberating journey, and it helps me tap into my leader within.

Further Inquiry

How have you naturally fostered community in your care-giving journey? What are you noticing about how people show up for you and your loved one(s)?

"This is the true joy of life, the being used for a purpose recognized by yourself as a mighty one; the being a force of nature instead of a feverish selfish little clod of ailments and grievances complaining that the world will not devote itself to making you happy.
I am of the opinion that my life belongs to the whole community, and as long as I live it is my privilege to do for it whatever I can."

–George Bernard Shaw, *Man and Superman*

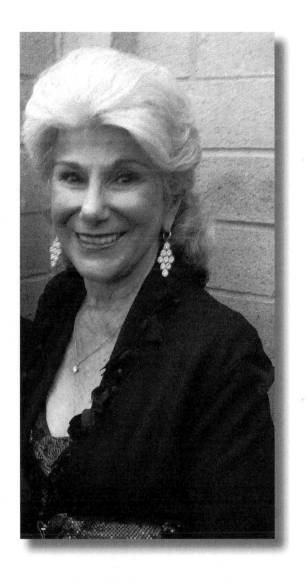

A visit to Michigan, on an upswing.

Brain Fog Can Be a Great Thing

One of you wonderful loved ones sent RAH a card with a quote from Winston Churchill: "If you're going through hell, keep going." And then another day, at the hotel, I was using a glass juice bottle to mix up my powdered Vitamin C, and I just happened to look at the inside of the bottle cap. Yep, again, the same quote. There are no accidents. It sure seems when I look in my mom's eyes (when they are open) that she is going going going, working hard at healing. Her eyes are so determined, even under sedation, and I wonder how much of this particular stint in ICU she'll remember. I hope not so much. RAH's throat is still swollen around the breathing tube, so they have not extubated yet. They'll try again sometime today. Sometimes the steroids take longer to work, according to the pulmonary specialist.

After that first year when it seemed like my mom's life was touch and go, like one more wrong move and she'd be dead at any time, my mom and I would have conversations about that year: her stay in ICU, all that happened during those months of recovering from surgery, starting the chemo regimen, other minor surgeries due to side effects of the original surgery and chemo, and a bunch of other details.

I was always relieved to hear her say she did not remember most of those initial fourteen days in the hospital. Phew! I remember feeling good that she had no memory of that time. I used to tell her that I was happy and grateful because it had been terrifying for me to watch her go through it, not able to keep her out of pain and discomfort.

This one conversation with my mom helped me understand things I previously knew nothing about. And it was the point when that old issue of "trust" started to tap me on the shoulder in new and different ways in order to bring lessons I needed to learn in my caregiving—both for my mom and for myself. I had to trust that 1) my mom was strong and capable enough to withstand this process, and 2) that I knew nothing about what it was truly like for her. After having conversations with her about it all, I became aware that the brain can protect the patient from some of the horrors they may experience as they are immersed in "patient-hood." It's like being a young child and falling down. You might have a scrape on your knee from the fall, but it's healing, and sometimes you don't even remember how you fell.

Further Inquiry

I hope this is also the case for your loved one and that you are able to relax just a bit in knowing they probably won't have the same experience as you when there's fear, worry, or anxiety involved. In its own way, it will all be okay. Is there a perspective you may not have considered yet?

"So it's true, when all is said and done, grief is the price we pay for love."

–E.A. Bucchianeri, *Brushstrokes of a Gadfly*

Use the Tools Out of Love

We are here in the ICU with RAH while she is napping peacefully after having been moved into a chair to change her position and get her blood and fluids circulating around. Still on the respirator, RAH is not too happy since she can't make a noise or speak, but we think she is also beginning to realize that she can't control the situation and that we are helping her take care of her main mission—to visualize peace, beauty, relaxation, and healing for herself, as we all are. The huge cartoon card arrived this morning from all her Michigan cousins, aunts, and uncles, and we set it at the foot of her bed. Thank you so much! We are getting her mail every day. It's going to be really fun to share it all with her and decorate her room with it.

We have chocolate truffle hearts at the foot of her bed with a note saying, "Happy Valentine's Day from Rosemary! Please help yourself." At this point, we are waiting for another test to see if she is getting the sufficient air leakage we have been waiting for around the tube in her airway so she can be extubated (please let it happen soon. Nicole won't leave until it happens, and I am getting tired of her toots in the hotel room—ha ha ha!). So, the word for today is patience. We are learning. It's a family trait: we are "do-ers." There are some lessons we learn along the journey: To be. To trust. To let go. To release. This is our visualization today.

Here's what I have come to realize now that I've got distance from the day-to-day mechanics and emotions of caregiving: Lifelong patterns of trying to control, fix, or manipulate circumstances to fit outcomes we are attached to (like my mom *not* having cancer and dying) are tough to shake. Instead of relaxing, trusting, and being still, I was used to being in motion.

Trusting the process, relinquishing control, and being patient with the everyday education I was receiving (unwillingly, mostly) was completely abnormal for me. It didn't fit the previous mindset I had adopted for my life. I came to embrace and normalize what I later called "the gifts of cancer." This was all a part of that gift pack I never really wanted to receive. And yet today, I am grateful that I was thrust into the new role as caregiver because it brought opportunities for me to learn more about my mom and, in turn, my own ways of being—whether they were constructive at the time or not. It was a part of my adult education, and I will always be appreciative of that, even though it meant my mom had to go eventually.

"Use the tools (don't let the tools use you)" is a mantra I've repeated in my business consulting practice over the years. I recently shared with a friend about how my mom prepared us for entrepreneurship our entire lives. She taught us to create systems and structures for maximum efficiency in ANY sort of business, as well as about the inherent challenges in growing a business.

Forget all the shiny-new objects. Go with what you know, create systems that serve you, keep them simple, and avoid getting caught up in every tool. Use and leverage tools that work. Leave the rest.

I remember nearing the fall of 2011, I thought for sure my mom would be a goner any minute. She was so weak and medically unstable. We couldn't care for her at home, so we had to search for a Skilled Nursing Facility close by. She stayed in one for more than a month. I was torn between leaving her there and having her at home, but we knew we couldn't help her, as she needed acute care. I was about to leave for Burning Man, and Nicole assured me that 1) Mom wouldn't die while I was gone (and my mom "promised" me as well), and 2) it was okay to take a break from writing daily journal entries (this was back in the days of me being "overly responsible"). Nicole also wrote updates of her own from time to time, thankfully. This support was invaluable for me.

I was able to go off to the Nevada desert for my annual pilgrimage that year and subsequent years knowing that life (and death) would unfold however it did, with or without me trying to be responsible and controlling every daily thing.

Further Inquiry

What gifts do you bring to your current challenges? I bet there are ways that your experiences in everyday life have informed and bolstered your experience in the caregiving journey you may be on today. It's important to do what you can tap in to naturally. And for what doesn't come naturally, out of love for yourself and your loved ones, be sure to tap in to your support team at various times.

"You can't heal the people you love.
You can't make choices for them.
You can promise that they won't
journey alone.
You can walk beside them.
But the journey is theirs."

–Laura Jean Truman

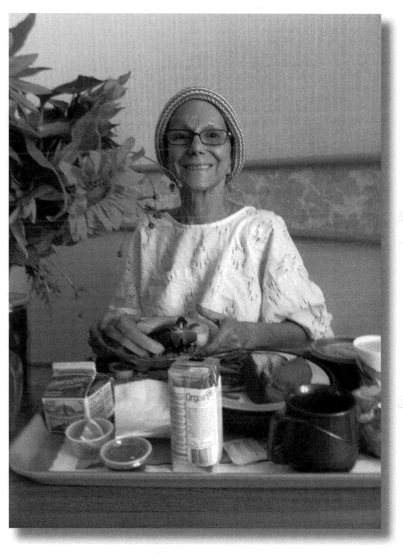

*The infamous "Happy Acres" stay, wasted away
and smiling through it.*

Laugh When You Can

Acomment on one of my journal entries from a dear friend who also helped us care for my mom gives a sense of how irreverent I can be, even in the most horrific of circumstances. It also encouraged me to continue to see and write about the humorous moments, which helps me.

> *These journal entries are better than TV or the Comedy Club!*
>
> *How you interpret for us in print the humorous moments in a day filled with challenges! It's beyond me! I feel so blessed to know you, RAH, and your amazing family of angels.*

Laugh when you can—anytime you can. I believe that laughter is medicine, and that gratitude heals. Even now, no matter what is happening that seems bleak, I try to insert some kind of perspective into the situation or circumstance that comes from a place of love, gratitude, humor, or (when I'm lucky) the trifecta—all three at once! **Normalize the funny stuff.** It may not always be appropriate or politically correct, but I'm beyond being concerned about what other people think of my approach. In fact, many of my mom's relatives appreciated my humor in the face of such heavy drama in our day-to-day lives.

And then, of course, no story about the funny side of cancer and treatment in a family system would be complete without mentioning poop. My mom fought the constipation. She hated being constipated, especially because her constitution had always been the envy of most. She could eliminate waste / take a shit any time, any place. On the regular, every day, no issues. Once the surgery and pharmaceutical drugs (including chemo) came into play, that was no longer the case. Part of her life after the cancer diagnosis was her inability to access that "regularity."

I often reminded her that six inches of her colon had been cut out, but that did not console her. She was mad about her state of constipation. She just wanted to take a dump like she used to without sitting on the toilet for hours and waiting (not so patiently). I didn't blame her a bit. I'd be mad too!

And believe me, she reported back every detail of her poops. She'd show us her estimated measurement using her thumb and index finger, or she'd say something like "it was a little pellet."

She made up language to describe her eliminations: poops, turds, BMs, moving bowels, pellets . . . it all became a part of our everyday life, and for some reason, even in the depths of the ugly dips, it was still amusing. So, we laughed when we could. Why is it that we turn into five-year-olds when we talk about poop? I'll never understand it, but I embrace it fully. The upshot in all this is that she (and we as her family caregivers) never had to endure a colostomy bag.

A family member once commented that they felt like they needed to comfort and console us because we were the ones dealing with this scary shit "on the ground," but instead, I was making them laugh, entertaining them with my humorous stories and perspectives on the grueling and uncomfortable circumstances we found ourselves in. This is how I normalized some of the tough stuff:

> *RAH is sitting on her "throne," waiting for her prince to come. (prince = poop)*
>
> *She gets all situated on the portable toilet (because she insists she needs to move her bowels), and all of a sudden I see her reaching forward to her bed, which is too far for her to reach, especially since she is so short that her feet are dangling and not firmly planted on the floor. I lean over to assist her because I think she might fall forward (and with the catheter and the IV still in her body, and the two drains leading out*

of her stomach into little dangling plastic bottles, this
would not have been pretty).

Mom: *"What are you doing?"*
Me: *"You look like you're going to fall off that thing.*
What are you reaching for?"
Mom: *"That sheet. It's not even and I am trying to*
straighten it out!"

Now, you would likely only relate to this if 1)
you are married to me (yes, I torture my dear, sweet
husband with "bed making by Lynn" ala my mom's
teachings), or 2) you have ever made a bed with my
mother. You see, we have a thing about bed making:
the sheets have to be perfectly even. A little over the
top? Yes. Hilarious in the hospital room setting? So
much yes!
Note: *My mom was a sheet-folding, bed-making ninja*
(yes, even with fitted sheets). Her bed was always like
a cloud palace. Always king-sized, fluffy, and fresh at
all times.

More humorous moments:
I had a **germaphobe "kit"** for every single visit or stay at any
hospital we found ourselves at. Gloves, homemade natural disinfectant spray and wipies, cleaning rags, towels for the floor to

set my laptop bag on (my mom's bags could usually fit in the tiny hospital room closet), paper towels, etc. If you are a germaphobe and are finding yourself in the germiest of all the places on earth, you are my people. And it's all going to be okay. We do what we have to do, and so what if we end up with a little more gear for such occasions? The minute we entered a new room or space, I sprayed and wiped down all the handles and drawer pulls . . . you get the idea. And all the while, I'd inhale my essential oils to ward off any cooties entering my body through my facial orifices. It had to happen. Every time. Nonnegotiable.

It's fun to remember **breaking rules** by bringing our own healthy food and candles into the hospital waiting room that very first night when we made ourselves a little fort using the chairs that were available. Of course, I sprayed down everything with my essential oil disinfectant spray and wiped all the armrests before I could relax a little. Okay, so there was no relaxing. Only waiting . . . waiting . . . playing that torturous waiting game in a hospital lobby. Good times (not).

During a **conversation about children,** RAH said, "All I had to do was put my shoes under the bed and I got pregnant—I had five!" I don't know why it struck us as so funny, but we laughed until we cried (and during those days, the two happened simultaneously at the drop of a hat). I had never heard that expression.

Mom **fell off the toilet seat** and into the trash bin (in the hospital room post-surgery). My sister caught her, so she wasn't injured. We laughed our asses off!

Cooked socks. When your little sister washes her socks in the hotel room sink and tries to dry them in the microwave, they burn and smell like roasted nuts. Now you know.

"Your breath smells." The minute my mom could finally talk after being extubated on Day 10, I went into the ICU to celebrate. I put my ear up to my mom's mouth so I could hear and hopefully understand her slurred speech. She whispered to me, "Your breath smells." I laughed to myself, grateful to her for providing some comic relief in the midst of her ICU recovery. For me, it meant my mom was coming back slowly and surely.

Further Inquiry

You will have moments when it's all too much and feels unbearably heavy. I encourage you to grasp on to any moments of mirth that you can muster. Write them down so you can recall them later, as I have often, and bring a smile through your tears of grief and longing. What are you noticing and what have you written down about the heavy moments and the light ones?

"Hey, sorry I'm late to the meeting. Society is crumbling and my body is failing me. Anyway, let's talk KPIs."

–@ryannoyance, Twitter

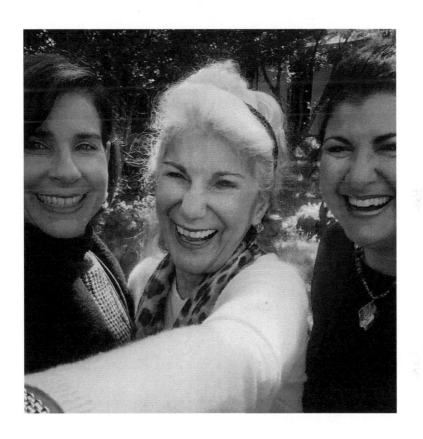

A favorite selfie: our mom with her "bookends."

Feeling It All

RAH is about the same and I can tell she is anxious to get that tube out and get on with her life. She gets so frustrated trying to talk and get messages across. She can only mouth words, which we cannot usually figure out. She wants to try and write, but she is partially sedated and so swollen that she can't hold a pen, much less write. I shared with her again tonight that there is nothing to do but try to relax, breathe, and rest up for tomorrow. I think it only made her more frustrated, which I can understand. She didn't want me to leave (I think). I tried to explain that she's getting really great care and that I had to go get some sleep so I could be back in the morning. She shook her head no. Luckily, RAH has a night nurse who seems really caring and sweet. He did a thorough check on all her vitals and her incision. It was extra hard to leave tonight, but I did my best to reassure her and waited until the very last minute. Her nurse

LYNN ABATÉ-JOHNSON

*assured me that he's keeping a close eye on her. He
calls her by her first name and explains all the things
he is doing to make her more comfortable. Big props
for that. Here's to a good night's rest for us all, and
especially RAH. Thank you for helping us be patient
while RAH's body does what it needs to do to heal.*

Navigating the guilt of watching my mom and not being able
to help her tore me apart. How could I possibly normalize this
situation? It wasn't normal; we weren't supposed to be going
through this. One notion that most people I know would never
want to discuss openly is the guilt that can accompany relief after
a family member dies. It's a double-edged sword. As a caregiver
and someone who hates to see someone they love suffer, it's a relief
that they no longer have to deal with the dis-ease. As a loving
daughter, at least for me, it was unfathomable I would be living
my life at a relatively young age without my mom.

You know when you have a tightening in your chest and a knot
in your stomach so big you can't breathe? I had to learn to make
peace with that feeling. The guilt I was experiencing was so real
for me, and so monumental. But the longer I stayed with it, the
less helpful I was for my mom. Thus, **I had to unlearn and relearn
my role as a strong daughter of a strong mother who was looking like she was going to leave the planet any minute. My new
role, whether I liked it or not, was to reassure her that she had
someone advocating for her at all times.**

I realize that we had the resources to be able to pull that off. We had helpers. When we needed breaks, we had extended family and friends we called to sit in for us. And we had systems in place to guide them. My heart goes out to those who, for whatever reason, don't have the resources that we did.

How do you come to grips with new roles and normalize the unimaginable circumstances and emotions that come up over time? Our new roles brought up more of the scary, unusual, never-before-conceived emotions and guilt, which all have their place. I look back now and recognize that it's critical to allow all of it. Give it a voice, speak the words, write the words, paint the pictures, make those playlists, move your body—help yourself to help yourself in making it okay to *NOT* be okay.

It was never OKAY for me, not by any stretch of the imagination, and yet I wasn't about to become a victim of my circumstances. My mom modeled that for me, so I found myself surrendering to her teaching and our lack of control.

Further Inquiry

How are you making sure you're feeling and releasing your emotions? Where do you feel it in your body when these emotions come up? I've noticed recently that my chest and my abdomen are the places I can feel my emotions. It's been helpful, and I hope you can tap in to this for yourself.

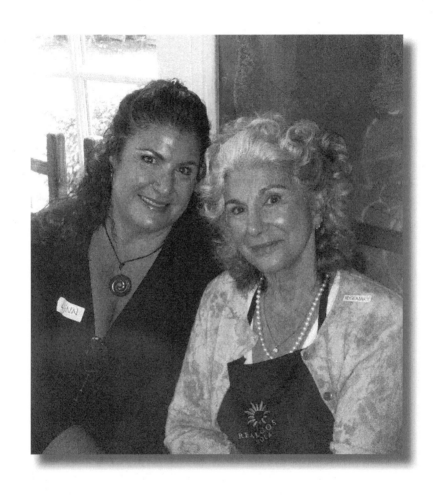

Grabbing every moment on the upswings.

LYNN ABATÉ-JOHNSON

"The world felt safer when my mother was here."

-@chelsohlemiller, Instagram

Expectations–It's a Setup

I am afraid to get a prediction from the doctors as to how long RAH will remain in the hospital. That "three days in the ICU" prediction went out the window eight days ago. It is not fun having that expectation in our heads. We keep thinking something is wrong, and we're teetering on losing our patience every day that the "garden hose" stays in RAH (her trachea has swollen up around it). So, for my part, don't give me any more predictions. Let's stick with the healthier version, shall we? How about one day at a time? Yeah, that works for me. Let's just stay in THIS moment. It's all we really have anyway. As long as RAH continues to make baby steps, I don't really care how long she is hospitalized. I'll deal with the germs/cooties. It'll all be okay. And the bonus is that she might just beat the crap out of cancer after all, even with such a scary diagnosis and surgery. We'll find out more about this when the expert panel meets with the tumor board, then gives us their complete results and recommended course of action.

"Oh, she'll probably be in ICU for about three days after surgery, and then she'll be released to a room." Ten days later, she was finally extubated and out of ICU. As a gentle note, don't believe everything you think or hear from the medical support team. Predictions are not only inaccurate at best, they also set up family caregivers/advocates for unnecessary fear and dread. It is all part of managing expectations that go with this territory. I realize (now) that it's unavoidable, but shit! I never thought I was an anxious person or at all susceptible to stress until all this started, and wow! I clung to every damn word and prediction the medical team even mentioned as a possibility. It was not great for my nervous system, or anyone else's, especially because I tried to keep the "freaking-the-F-out" look off my face when I was around my mom, siblings, nieces, and nephews. It's hard to fake that. If you know, you know.

I quickly learned over the first few months that I needed to manage my own expectations in the face of any type of "prediction," especially when it came to the timing of a person's system to recover and heal. There's no point in investing heavily in any educated guesses or estimates. I created mantras for myself in these cases after being disappointed and emotionally rattled when the timing didn't line up as expected. I would say things to myself like: "It takes what it takes" and "Trust Mom's mind, body, spirit to do what they need to do to help her through this" and "You don't have control here." Trust. That's a big one for me. I didn't realize that trusting was abnormal for me until I was faced with all the nuances I could not control. Looking back, it's one of the most important things I wish I would have had back then . . . trust.

Further Inquiry

What expectations are you holding on to? What prompts or mantras can you create to help navigate through thwarted expectations?

"Transformation is not about creating a new life, it's about seeing life in a new way."

–@anabel.vizcarra, Instagram

Perspectives and Relationships

Tonight, my husband, Corey, got to come see RAH on his way to work. He said, "Wow, she seems so weak," to which I replied, "That's nothing. You should have seen her four or five days ago. She's made amazing progress since then." It reminded me that perspective is everything, especially in this case. RAH can now do a (very modified) bridge pose in bed by digging her feet in and propping herself up with her arms just enough for her nurse to scoot a towel under her bootie. Her muscles will remember what to do. She just needs to retrain them little by little. So we are grateful for baby steps, deeper and deeper belly breaths, and visiting husbands/sons-in-love. By the way, RAH is really enjoying all your messages, cards, love notes, emails. Nicole has done a great job of catching her up on all the love flowing to her from you and is decorating her room with all your photos, artwork, cards, and flowers. Thank you for being on this journey with us.

Oh, the sweetness of the power of perspective. I remember this part of the extended hospital stay "roller coaster" so well. Not only was I aghast at the level of germs and extra fluid I was around, I was also trying to view this change in my life with a fresh perspective. I hadn't seen Corey in a while, and he loved my mother so much. He was *way* more patient with her than I ever could be. And she loved him too. There's a beautiful bond that will always remain in our hearts; it's the relationship that grew over time. My mom always saw the best in Corey, and he saw the best in her.

The year before my mom's diagnosis, Corey and I had hit a wall in our marriage. It was quite a doozy. We got help from a psychologist who really made an impact on us, both individually and in our relationship.

Although things worked out (we chose to stay married after all the ups and downs we experienced that year), I grappled with being my mom's caregiver and Corey's wife at the same time. I wasn't sure our marriage would withstand my long absences and full attention on her. And yet, there he was, showing up at the hospital on his way to the airport (which wasn't really on his way, but it was close enough. He wanted to see her for himself as well as visit me).

So, there was his perspective, seeing her so weak and unlike herself, and mine, seeing how she had progressed in the two weeks since her surgery. And then there was another perspective I held, which was how rock-solid Corey was in prioritizing his love and care for my mom like I was (and in his own way).

I remember being so insecure about my marriage at that time. Would it survive this bump? Would I be able to be fully present with my husband during the scariest, all-hands-on-deck times when my mom needed me to be present? Was I replaceable? (That question was difficult to come to terms with. I wanted to fix everything. I wanted to make it all better, and I wanted to be the one to do it for my mom and for my husband.) How much responsibility did I have, longing to be in both places at the same time?

I remember always feeling torn, and what I realize now was that I was making up scenarios. I was constantly having conversations with myself, and I now see that this was something I was not alone in doing. This is my opportunity to **help normalize fear, guilt, and those feelings of being torn** between my responsibilities of being both a daughter and a spouse. I am thankful that Corey and I are still together, and the aftermath of losing my mom, his mother-in-love, is that we seem to have made it over that particular life hurdle while learning a lot about ourselves, each other, and our relationship as we continue navigating a new life and a new world together.

I have since learned that trusting myself and my loved ones, as well as the support system I've created over time, is key in my own leadership journey. Trust. There's that word again. I wasn't thinking of it at that time. I see it so much clearer now, with years of distance and some personal growth because of the assistance I've invested in over these years, including hiring a personal coach. Back then, I was often simply going through the motions to get through each day, tending to my mom and my family as best I could. I navigated being a wife, daughter, big sister, aunty, friend. (I don't even remember being in touch with many of my friends on a deep level during those years except for the ones who generously volunteered to help us care for my mom.)

For as long as I walk this planet, I will look back on that tumultuous time with gratitude for the trust I was able to develop and continue to hone. Even more important for me is to be responsible for my own inner power and wisdom. I must listen to my inner leader. I learned more about myself through those years than I realized, because when I was immersed in caring for my mom, I couldn't see how I was *being*. All I could see was my *doing*. More perspective.

Further Inquiry

What or who can you tap in to in order to get insights you may be missing by being so close to your current circumstances? Have you considered working with a coach? Remember also that your inner leader is there. Tap in to them.

"To describe my mother would be to write about a hurricane in its perfect power."

–Maya Angelou, *I Know Why the Caged Bird Sings*

Protect the Sleep!

Five times. Yep, we were up five times during the night after the movie ended at 12:30 a.m. (of course, I took a little nap during the movie since I've seen it a hundred times. The Princess Bride—a classic and funny movie). RAH had to make several trips to her "throne" throughout the night. After that, in a desperate attempt to help her sleep, I turned on my noise maker, which helped her fall back asleep for a couple hours. All in all, not much consistent sleep happened. Oh well. There are other nights.

The sleep! I remember all the nights of being up and down. Neither my mom nor I were really great at falling back to sleep once we woke up, and we never learned the art of napping. I loved seeing my mom do any little thing that showed she was feeling somewhat "normal." Reading was a big one. She was a voracious reader. She'd devour fiction novels, except when she wasn't feeling well. There were periods of time when no reading happened at all, so when she finally picked up a novel again in between bouts with the dis-ease and the side effects of the meds and chemotherapy, I did a little happy dance in my heart. Over those cancer years (and especially since then), I realized I was playing those kinds of mental games in my head—watching my mom for signs she was feeling better and going to make it through whatever valley we were in. I was extremely attached to her well-being. If she felt good, I felt good. If she felt like shit, I started spinning emotionally and losing sleep over all the impending doom and gloom. It was warranted, expected, and natural that I processed in *my* way. No one else processed exactly how I did. I actually appreciated the different styles of coping we displayed as a family collective. I have never been a mom, so I didn't have the wisdom to understand that I had to look at the whole picture, something my sister Nicole reminded me to do. Nicole was able to relate our mom's dis-ease to times when her kids were sick and recovering. So she coached me with reassurance like "you have to look at the big picture and not just focus solely on the current crisis."

The issue I had was that everything became so extreme for me. The emotions I had spinning around my mom's every move, her every waking (and even resting) moment, determined how my days and nights went. I learned over the cancer years to develop a keener sense of how to be with my emotions and how to process them better and better (never perfectly, of course), as well as how to detach with love.

I felt what my mom felt, bottom line. And it wasn't only empathically. Because this woman birthed me and raised me, I sometimes felt like I was her. I felt everything at a cellular level. I remember a specific conversation we had one day while sitting quietly in the hospital room:

> Me: "I'm so sorry, Mom."
> Mom: "For what?"
> Me: "That this is happening to you. If I could switch places with you, I would."
> Mom: "No! Don't even think that!"

It was devastating for her to think of losing any of her children. Yet I know that if the roles had been reversed, she would have handled it in her own unique way. She would have also done everything possible to be sure she exhausted every avenue, every healing modality, in the hope of saving *my* life.

In fact, during those times when I would get so furious at her for not drinking enough water or eating shit that the cancer fed on (sugar), I would remind her that if our roles were reversed, she would never let me get away with that kind of stuff. She'd hover over me like I hovered over her and exhaust herself the way I did, physically and emotionally. It was not a good look for me, nor was it healthy for her to have me getting on her case about that stupid shit (and in hindsight, I can say it was "stupid shit," but back then it was literally *life* or *death* in my narrow caregiver view).

As I was concerned about my mom getting her sleep while her body was fighting the cancer and trying to live, I lost my grip on my own sleep. Everything was a major contributor to my sleeplessness during those years: my mom's lack of water, her sugar consumption, my guilt that she was sick and I wasn't, the conflict we had over any little thing. Ugh! My emotions spun through my head every night, all night. I had plenty to spin about, of course. It was all valid, but it did not belong in my brain when it was time to sleep. Still, it was always there. I did a *terrible* job of managing this area of my life back then, and I am now extremely protective of it. If I'm not sleeping well, I go back to what I know typically works well for me so that I can be well rested enough to function optimally for both myself and for others in my life today. Sleep is precious. Perhaps you need extra hydration, or to try herbal remedies, take your eyes off digital screens, have your hormones checked, "wind down" from earlier stimulation—it's all worth trying until you are able to balance that part of your life. Protect your sleep as much as possible.

Further Inquiry

How are you caring for yourself at this moment, especially in the area of guarding your sleep?

"One day you will tell your story of how you overcame what you went through and it will be someone else's survival guide."

–Brené Brown

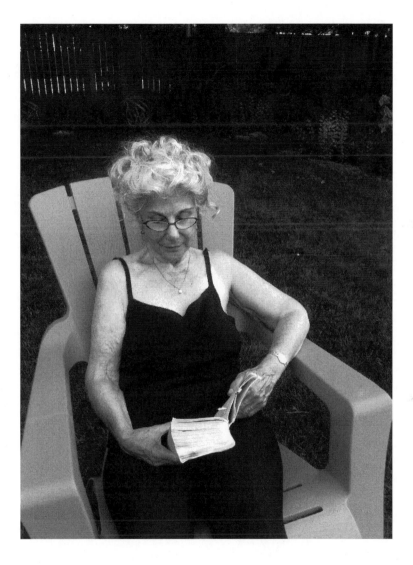

Summertime reads in my Sonoma Valley backyard.

What Is Normal Anyway?

We got *the news today that RAH now has her chemo-therapy assignment from the clinical trial committee. Here's the layout, for those who are in "the know" and care to have the details:*

Paclitaxel 135 mg/m2 IV over 3 hours on Day 1

Cisplatin 75 mg/m/2 IP on Day 2

Paclitaxel 60 mg/m2 IP on Day 8

(repeated every 3 weeks for 6 cycles)

Bevacizumab 15 mg/kg IV during chemotherapy cycles 2–6, and then cycles 7–22 after completion of chemotherapy.

Total treatment time is supposed to last for 15 months. RAH will have her IV (clavicle) and IP (abdominal) ports placed soon by her surgeon. In the meantime, we'll be lining up our schedule to get RAH down to the treatment center. At first, we'll get the "lay of the land" ourselves and accompany RAH en force, then later, we'll accept some offers from local friends to do some driving. Everyone has been so kind and generous. We are so grateful. Now we need to fatten up RAH a bit before it all begins.

My purpose in sharing this information is not to compare it to anyone else's experience or to get too clinical; however, I think it provides better context woven into my mom's journey. My mom opted into an aggressive clinical trial. Her surgeon was the chief investigator, so he had a stake in helping to extend her life if this approach was to work for her.

Every step of this journey was an exercise in curious exploration, navigating what seemed surreal. My ideas of "normal" were completely thrown out the window. In the case of getting my mom's chemotherapy assignment for the clinical trial we were about to embark upon, I found myself grasping for any sense of "normal" I could muster up. Without a frame of reference, and no prior experience, what was normal for me at the time was to think critically while grappling with much emotion, stress, and anxiety.

These were the components of my everyday life at the time that became "normal," and they started to become unmanageable because they were manifesting in my physical condition. I wasn't sleeping well, and I was sugar-bingeing and packing on my own inflammation as the cancer was blowing up my mom's body. As for my mom, the treatment only heightened her inflammation, so there was daily management of the side effects of the cancer, the treatment, and the stress on my mom and her body. It was almost like a circus where juggling and jumping from event to event became our new normal. It was no fun at all. Everything was unpredictably trauma inducing.

And this is where I get to reassure caregivers, once again, that being in this challenging life-or-death circumstance is navigable beyond what you can see in front of you. I have reflected on this in the years since my mom died—how I came to terms with my mom being in pain and eventually taking her final breath. I had the luxury of time that so many others do not, given a multitude of unique circumstances. I can't say that I got used to the reality of my mom's struggle, but I can say that I gradually learned to accept the things I could not control. I later learned through my grief counseling sessions with the hospice counselor that I had adopted a mechanism they call "anticipatory grief." When we are in the throes of daily circumstances, it often seems as if we are buried in a dark hole without a light to guide us. As the days, weeks, months, and years passed for me, I was able to gain more perspective by practicing acceptance as a mindset, even when I was having "arguments" with myself to do the opposite—to NOT accept it. I know you will find ways to adapt and adjust as well, if you haven't done so already. We get to choose how we view every detail of every challenge. I realize it's easier said than done when you are still in it, however.

Further Inquiry

What has your current situation (today, right now) been teaching you that you didn't realize before?

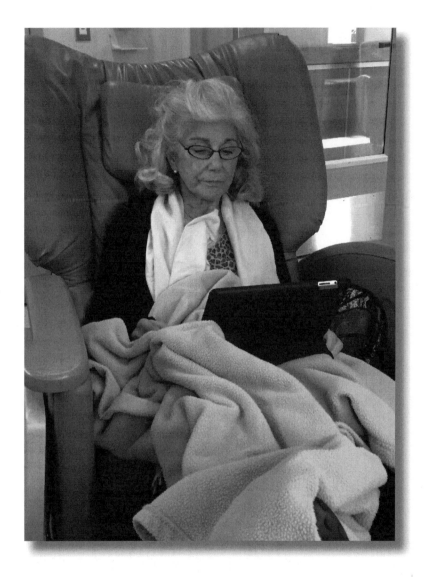

Taking care of business in pearls and cashmere during chemo.

LYNN ABATÉ-JOHNSON

"Being deeply loved by someone gives you strength, while loving someone deeply gives you courage."

–Lao Tzu

Control Freaks Unite!

RAH is through her first day of chemo, and so far, so good. She's in great spirits, and she's coming up with some very funny one-liners. In the car on the way in, Nicole asked RAH how she was feeling, to which she replied, "Fine, and how are YOU feeling?" RAH's first entry in her new chemo journal is: "I am here. Life is good. They have treats!" There is a kitchen here for the patients stocked with some not-so-desirable-but-still-desirable things like cheesy crackers and candy bars. RAH added, "I'll have to advise them on the good stuff—better yet, I'll bring my own."

Later that day, my journal entry continues:

Energizer Bunny is home! RAH is whizzing around this evening, albeit a bit more slowly than normal (it's more a WAS than a WHIZ at this point, but that's temporary).

RAH: *"I think I need to lie down. My tummy hurts."* *This feisty little lady knows her body, so this is a great time to support her in getting ready for an early night to bed since we have an even earlier call tomorrow morning. We need to be up and out of the house (to deal with the fun rush-hour traffic).*

Control and the lack of it. This was a big lesson for me while supporting my mom to the best of my ability and also learning to be more patient and trusting throughout the process. It often seemed like time flew by, and yet the days seemed so long, especially when my mom wasn't feeling well. This became a paradox that defined the construct of time for me. Impatient people will be tested throughout their caregiving journey. If I could have normalized being out of control (and naturally impatient), it would have helped me cope on the days that were painful for my mom, and thus, me.

Happily, even though I was having a difficult time relinquishing control, I was able to create lists and tracking charts. On chemotherapy days, for example, I knew our emotions would be in full force, so I had a list in front of us to be sure we had all the comfort items and practical things we might need for long days away, both on the road and at the cancer center.

- Favorite pillow
- Neck pillow (yes, all the different pillows!)
- Blanket
- Cozy hat and gloves
- Fitted sheet for covering the foldout chair
- Medical notebook
- Chargers for electronics
- High-impact snacks
- Healthy bottled water to refill insulated cup with straw
- Toiletries
- Disinfectant spray (natural, of course)
- Wipes
- Change of underwear
- Change of clothes
- Slippers
- Heating pad
- Current book
- Music-playing device with headphones
- Extra batteries
- Reading glasses
- Eye drops

We had lists for the car, the chemotherapy room, my mom's purse, a tote bag, and the rolling suitcase. It was absolutely a sight to see. It also made a big difference in my mom's comfort level, and ours, while delving into such unknown territory.

Further Inquiry

If you feel as if you need to control something, make a list. Maybe you already have one. Now that I've been through our journey, I can look back and say, "Yep, I wasn't great at letting go of control, but I was good at making lists." And maybe that will have to be enough for you too. When you're in the middle of the chaos, sometimes "changing" won't be an option, and you leaning on your strengths will be what helps. What strengths do you have that are helping with your current caregiver situation? Pat yourself on the back for that.

"This is hope:
I do not know what is next
but I am catching a glimpse
of something beautiful.
I am finding
grace-lined strength
even though I wasn't sure
I could make it this far.
I am finding flickers of hope
as radiant and immeasurable as the stars.
And even though new fears still find me
and the ground feels shaky
beneath my feet,
I will trust that hope is still real
even if it seems far beyond me.
And maybe
after everything
I am not as lost
as I feel,
and even here
there is room to breathe
rest
heal."

–@morganharpernichols, Instagram

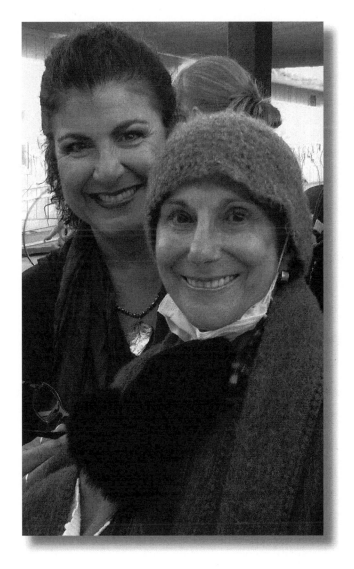

Seventy-nine pounds of strength through a scary time of cachexia.

Food Obsessed

Day two of chemo. Again, so far, so good (we know it may get really rough after this, but we're enjoying a relative "honeymoon" for now). RAH has relaxed, laughed (she cracks up over her own jokes), and entertained the nurses and the doctor. We shared our snacks with the medical oncologist, introducing him to cashew, walnut, and macadamia nut butters, as well as some sprouted crackers. We also shared organic pear slices and bananas around the room. Then we sent the doctor off to the hospital for rounds with RAH's favorite staple protein drink, which he said would be his lunch.

Later:

RAH: *"What I really need is a delicious, fresh-made donut!"*

Where does she come up with this stuff? Monday night after surgery, all she wanted was a root beer. The day after her big surgery, in the ICU with a "garden hose" down her throat, she wanted 7-Up with ice. She NEVER eats donuts, let alone has a craving for one. Right after she asked for the donut, the nurse walked in and said, "Would a cupcake do?" and offered us an entire tray of cupcakes. RAH just about split a gut laughing, then took one.

RAH: "I think I'll eat my salad now, because otherwise, I won't have my cupcake left." One delicious salad with homemade dressing and hard-boiled egg coming up!

How do we navigate an obsession with food under these new circumstances? For longer than I care to admit here, I often found myself obsessed with, and hanging on to, every bite my mom would take. For a family of foodies, I guess it wasn't out of character; however, in my particular case, as someone who has used food the way some use alcohol or drugs, or anything else to escape circumstances with the illusion of comfort, it wasn't a healthy focus for me. My insistence on getting my mom to eat, plus listing every morsel that went into her body (like some mothers do with a new baby) became obsessive, and for good reason.

I used salt and sugar (in various forms) to comfort myself. I thought that if I could enjoy a sweet coffee drink or my favorite salty/crunchy snack (think nachos), I would conjure up the feelings of comfort I was craving. I also used my mother's dislike of me being fat against her. I'd say stupid shit to her like "If you don't eat, I'm going to eat it, and more, then gain back the fifty-three pounds I just lost!" Oof, I hate even admitting I'd say things like this to try and manipulate her into stuffing her own face.

My mom was the original foodie influence in my life. She made gourmet meals on a shoestring budget. No matter how poor my parents were with five children to feed, my mom put it all together in the form of healthy, nutritious meals. She could "make a dollar stretch" as they used to say.

During the cancer years, I thought I could manipulate, threaten, cajole, or blackmail her into eating. Obviously, these tactics didn't work. It was based on such bullshit—my own bullshit about my self-care, my caring for her, and the impact of the family dis-ease at hand, all of which has informed my leadership journey over all these years: how I lead from within and how I lead in the systems I'm a part of. Having people in my corner who call me on my bullshit is key. I highly recommend finding those people who care enough to lovingly call you out when you are "feeding" yourself bullshit.

I'll say this about my food obsession: It seemed normal for me, since it was already an issue and an addiction. I suppose it's no different than any other addiction. Something catastrophic happens, it becomes a trigger, and we succumb to our addictions in order to make life seem "normal" when it's far from that.

Today, I'm so much healthier than I was during the cancer years and in more ways than just my physical health. I have learned to use food and not let it use me. Mostly. I still practice getting a handle on emotional triggers that can lead me to eat for comfort (or any other reason than hunger). I am training myself to ask whether I'm hungry for food or something else like attention, acknowledgment, belonging, or connection.

I've created space that I didn't have before my mom died (and if I'm honest, during my entire teen and adult years). The space I give myself now comes in the form of a healthy pause. Rather than impulsively or habitually grabbing something to put into my mouth, I hit that pause button in my head and got curious. What am I hungry for in this moment? It's an inquiry that really makes a difference. I'm probably in the fittest condition I've been in since before life circumstances piled on the unhealthy coping mechanisms.

The impact of having the space and forethought to get curious about how I treat myself is that I can look back on all the years I was in the "thick of it"—before and during the cancer years— using food to cope with life's circumstances. And when I reflect,

I am filled with gratitude that I was able to correct the course of my life and create a healthier trajectory for whatever remaining years I have on this earth. I'd like to think that I'm also in a better position to help others along their self-leadership journeys by being very honest about where I was and where I am headed. I attribute my healthier perspectives to the communities I've generated over the years, seeking out those who understand and love me through the many changes and painful growth spurts I've been fortunate enough to navigate. The fact that I've published this book is a testament to the circle of people who I've chosen to help guide me, hold me, and see me in ways I had not been able or willing to see myself.

I used to think that being fiercely independent was the way to go. I've learned since those cancer years that I was missing so much in terms of my personal development and leadership journey.

"Going it alone" was never the answer. Getting curious and asking for support is where true self-leadership thrives.

Further Inquiry

If you allow yourself a moment to pause and reflect, what kinds of habits are you naturally falling in to and how can you evolve what's happening into healthier ways of coping, even if only for a minute or two?

"Are you okay, or are you the eldest daughter?"

–@wolfgini, Instagram

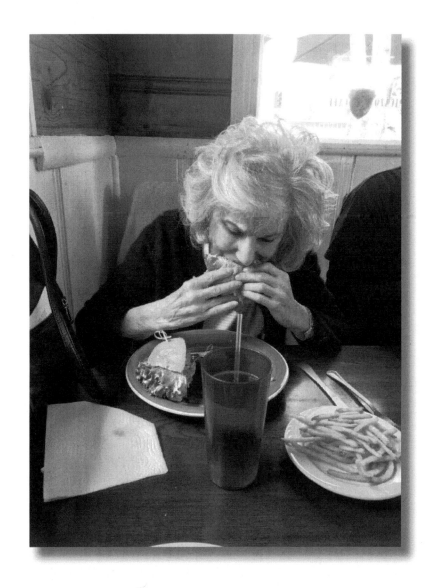

Yes to eating! Always a joy to behold.

LYNN ABATÉ-JOHNSON

Pause and Patience

RAH's pain management is getting better, although it's continuing to be a bit of a roller coaster.

Between healing from surgery, missing some "parts," lacking physical movement, and getting her digestive system back on track (plus the added little "party" going on in her kidneys), RAH's body is reeling, as you can imagine. Last night at the hospital, we ran into one of her fabulous nurses who said that many people younger than RAH who have had this extensive surgery do not do as well as she is, especially this soon afterward. So, we continue to make the best of a situation none of us ever expected, let alone asked for. Of course, philosophically speaking, one might argue that this journey was meant for us. And, indeed, it has had its lessons along the way. Like how to pause. How to stay in the moment—the present. Take one day at a time, literally. How to practice, practice, practice patience. And tolerance. And trust. Did I mention patience? Those of you who know us well, especially "us" being the women in our family, get it. These are lessons we don't always welcome, and yet we are (mostly) willing to stay open and heal right along with each other. Healing takes many forms. This journey is all about that, and more.

Have you ever wondered about the roles we play in a family, especially when a loved one is in need? We all approach challenges differently, and I've been on a steep learning curve.

Things like pausing, being still, being curious, having trust, and asking for help are now more than mere concepts in my life. They have all become cornerstones in the community I've been building. I've realized more and more that we all need each other and that it's not a sign of weakness to ask for what you need, including acknowledgment. I understood it on an intellectual level before my mom died and have since made it a priority to practice these new cornerstones in my life.

My family dynamic (growing up with two strong cultural backgrounds) generally dictated that "fighting is fatal." If you argued or had some differences with family members or friends, it was perfectly natural (and even encouraged) to cut them off. This was hardwired into me from a young age, so it's going to take the rest of my life to practice being openhearted and to stand in curiosity, love, and passion for what I believe in, while also opening myself up to new ideas, approaches, and perspectives. It's been very uncomfortable at times, in the years since my mom's death, to pause, assess, and choose (based on my personal judgment) where to turn and how to proceed. As I say, it's a practice, and there's no "there" to arrive at. However, I will say that as uncomfortable and challenging as this practice has been so far, it's better than the alternative. And, I have all the privilege our system and culture have assigned me. In my acknowledgment of my privilege, I'm also keenly aware that I grapple with previous misconceptions about myself, my identity, and my place in the world today. Ironically, as I continue my own personal transformation throughout these years, I also acknowledge that families, especially those with a strong matriarch, can be affected when that matriarch is no longer the "glue" that connects them. I have observed other families who have experienced the death of a parent or parents, where "cracks" in the family system can become more pronounced. My family has been no exception. Our dynamics have shifted, and in some cases dramatically, over the years. It's an ever-changing landscape of relationships, and it's neither good nor bad. It simply is. Again, patience, acceptance, and pausing with curiosity are all tools I've been developing in my own life over time, and I will continue to do so. My responsibility is to continue to care for myself so that I can have an overflow of energy and resources with which to support those I care about.

I appreciate the Ram Dass assertion that we are all just "walking each other home." That resonates with my empathic warrior soul. It grounds me.

And so, you will be okay through all you are navigating if you can take pauses. Be super loving and gentle with yourself as you pass through the dark times; be present when you have "wins" along the way. It's all part of our journeys, in relationship with ourselves, first and foremost.

Further Inquiry

What are you curious about at this moment? What comes up for you when you pause to consider it? How have your family dynamics come into play in these moments?

"After all my years working with the dying and the grieving, I have found that in this lifetime, the ultimate meaning we find is in everyone we have loved. Your loved one's story is over. For unknown reasons, their time on earth has drawn to a close, but yours continues. I can only invite you to be curious about the rest of the story of your life."

–David Kessler, *Finding Meaning: The Sixth Stage of Grief*

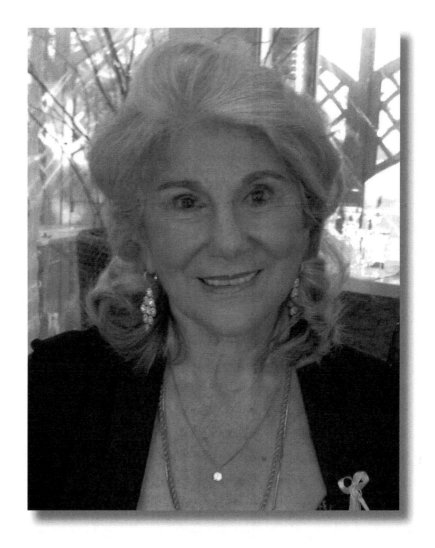

Elegant and poised on a visit to Michigan.

Courage in the Face of Fear

Yes, folks, we are back in the tender loving care of one of the local hospitals. RAH was admitted during the night and there was little-to-no sleep happening because of all the testing, poking, and conversations about RAH's journey up until this point (it's always a different staff, and I remember in most visits to the emergency departments, the staff didn't know what chemo thrash looked like, so they'd pull out "end-of-life" paperwork for us to fill out before they'd see or examine her). Of course, RAH's doctors have been consulted, especially her oncologist, who is keeping abreast of every twist and turn so that he can adjust the next cycle of chemo, if necessary, as well as guide us through what he says is pretty normal "stuff" for the first cycle of chemo under RAH's belt. The short of it is that RAH's white blood cell count is very low, something that was predicted. Luckily, a dear family member who had medical training caught it while caring for RAH last night in discovering that RAH's temp was above normal.

RAH's quote for the day: "I'm perfectly healthy except for the cancer."

Because one of my significant reasons for sharing my story is to help others feel like they have the company of someone who has been in a similar situation, this particular period of our journey is one I will always remember. It was my first time learning about white blood cells and their levels, as well as what it looks like and what it entails to recover from a white blood cell "crash." I was with my mom day and night in the hospital room, and everyone had to be fully geared up to even walk into that room: booties on shoes, head coverings, masks, and gowns. This went on for a full week. I think I panicked at first because of my aversion to germs, especially hospital germs. But I was able to "steel myself" as one of my sisters advised me to do back when our mom was in ICU (when I almost passed out from seeing her so lifeless for those ten days). It was much more important that my mom have an advocate there 24/7 than to worry about my idiosyncrasies and phobias.

This was a harrowing week in the hospital, and I remember it vividly. I found courage I didn't know I had in that I never imagined that I'd be in a hospital room with my mom for a week or more, with all my preconceived notions of "hospital life" (exposure to germs, lack of sleep, etc.), plus always stepping up to be an advocate for my mom.

Ah, my germ phobia. **I've spoken about normalizing fears and anxiety.** This is one of many I had to figure out while we were navigating the ins and outs of emergency visits and hospital stays. Yuck! I've always held the belief that hospitals are germy, and I know that people can also get wonderful care and healing there. It's a double-edged sword, to be sure. This played into my growing sense of "something's wrong here" and this is not "normal." How did I normalize it for myself? All my germ-fighting tips and tricks came into play, and I felt pretty confident most of the time that as long as I had my natural disinfectants, plenty of chuck pads, and gloves to avoid touching too many germs while I wiped down the room every time we were admitted, then we'd be okay. I was very committed to dealing with whatever my mom's body was doing at any given time without worrying about some random, opportunistic infection or extra dis-ease cropping up while we were on the hospital premises.

If you are at all squeamish or prone to germaphobia like I was (and still am, to an extent), you can learn ways to mitigate what you can control while letting the rest go. It's very possible to control more than we think, even when it comes to physical surfaces in a hospital setting. I started learning to release my fears, which gave way to the courage it took for me to stay the course when it was necessary.

Further Inquiry

Where have you found courage recently in your journey?

What are you learning to let go of in the process?

"When you devote yourself to more rest, your NO becomes more loving and courageous. You embrace NO as the foundation to your most sacred YES."

–Octavia Raheem, *Pause, Rest, Be*

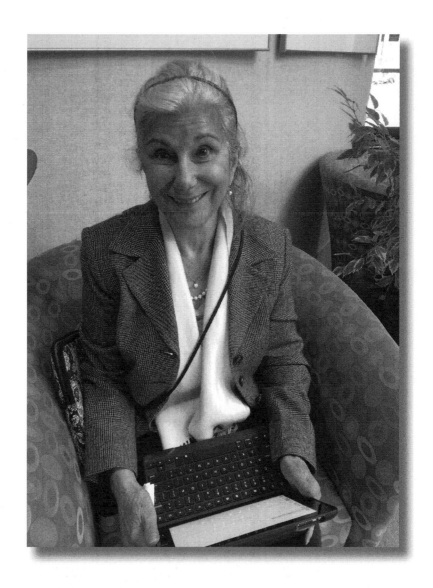

The original entrepreneur in my life getting it all done.

LYNN ABATÉ-JOHNSON

Through Strangers' Eyes

This little mama can saw logs! Okay, this is going to be an interesting night in more ways than one. RAH is fast asleep, since about 9:45 p.m., with no pain keeping her awake, and snoring like you wouldn't believe. She also weighed in 2 lbs more than she did last Wednesday at chemo, so that's exciting news. Notice we are focusing (as usual) on the positives, and (as usual) we are extremely grateful for the wonderful, competent, caring hospital team. In fact, this evening, RAH's emergency department nurse, the one she really connected with and who stuck with her the last time we were here, came up to say hi (and to check on RAH) shortly after she reported in for work. She is so sweet with RAH, giving her lots of love and nurturing. She was with RAH most of the night last night when we arrived at the ED and then admitted us to a room around 5 a.m. This nurse complimented RAH by telling her that she sure raised her children right. (Okay, okay, so all that strict parenting DID pay off, and I am the first to admit that I am all the better for it, I guess.)

Now, through this experience and journey, we get to see how RAH has touched so many lives in her five short years in Sonoma since her retirement, and in the many years that led up to this moment. There are so many beautiful people who are pulling and praying for her. That, in itself, is a huge gift for all of us.

For all the years growing up with my strict, strong, sometimes intimidating little mama, I was gifted with perspective in my later years. I didn't appreciate who she was when she was making me and my four siblings pick 100 weeds (each) in the yard every Saturday before we could go do fun things with our friends. The math = 500 weeds every Saturday!

I didn't appreciate my friends thinking she was so "cool" when she was forcing me to do other household chores. And so, it became a regular practice throughout those cancer years to see my mom through the eyes of others. Her natural charisma, kindness, enthusiasm, and pragmatism during the toughest of days, weeks, months—I now saw it all in a different light as the adult version of myself on the front lines advocating and caring for her. Those are moments I will always treasure. The realization of the impact my mom had on her community and her world was a gift that kept giving, and to this day, I tear up whenever I read one of the comments from our online journal, especially after she died. Seeing my mom's beautiful nature through other's eyes is truly an ongoing part of the comfort inside of my personal grief journey.

Further Inquiry

What realizations about your loved one have you made during your own journey together? What do you appreciate learning from them? You may have to dig deep. I realize it's not easy. However, for me, it has been worth it. Especially because I know that I was an asshole to my mom when I was a young and unappreciative teen, taking her for granted. This is the gift of hindsight and having gone through a cancer journey together.

"I would say that compassion for our parents is the true sign of maturity."

—Anaïs Nin, *The Diary of Anaïs Nin Volume 5*

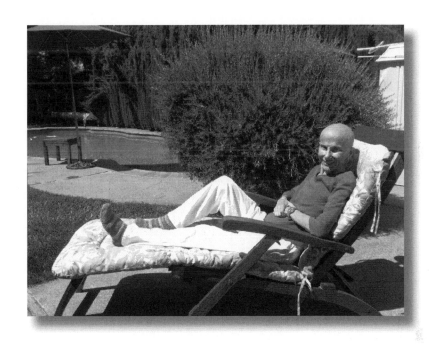

Poolside Vitamin D at my Sonoma Valley home.

Call Me by My First Name

RAH had a great day and evening overall. Her import-ant blood levels are up and getting better each day, so all the specialists who have seen her are encouraged and are keeping a close watch on daily results. She is going to bed feeling happy, positive, and ready to get a good night's sleep. The nursing staff has finished up their work for the evening with instructions to please leave RAH alone for the entire night. There are to be no vitals taken or anything else except to turn off any alarms or if I ring their buzzer.

We post a sign on her door during every hospital stay. We keep it as big, bold, and simple as possible. It provides basic info that anyone can access in the middle of the night if they happen to miss it in the darkened room:

My name is _____.

Please call me by my first name.

My date of birth is _____.

I am here for _____ **treatment
(or** _____ **procedure).**

**Please do not wake me for anything that is not
immediately vital. Let me rest.**

Doctor's name: _____.

My children's names and phone numbers:

_____

_____

_____

_____

*It has worked great the past two nights, rewarding
RAH with a full night's sleep, which is making a big
difference, especially considering how exhausted and
depleted she was when we arrived in the ED. RAH
was feeling great this evening, and being remarkably
alert, she asked me to take her for a walk. And then,
a couple hours later, she asked to get up, brush and
floss her teeth in preparation for bedtime, and then go*

for yet ANOTHER WALK. She said it was her fourth walk of the day. I didn't look it up on the log to verify, but I believe it (sometimes RAH forgets stuff, which is completely normal for what she is experiencing).

RAH has already done ten of her "suck-toy" exercises this morning, and it's not even 8:00 a.m.!
Me: *"Mom, use your tummy muscles."*
RAH: *"I used those all up yesterday."*
Ha ha ha. She is hilarious.
Then, while RAH and I were preparing to apply hand lotion to ourselves, she said:
"Let me roll up your sleeves for you."
Me: *"You're never going to stop mothering me, are you?"*
RAH: *"Nope. When I am ninety, you'll be sixty."*

So much joy is found in these moments, and they continue to help my heart heal as I look back on funny and tender moments through all the times we were alone together in various locations (hospitals, doctors' offices, at home).

Realizing the similarities and the differences between my mom and me, and especially times when I was challenged by her, **helped me come to grips with the twists and turns every relationship holds.**

I used to joke with my mom by saying, "I inherited all your best qualities, Mom!" We'd have a laugh. I think she agreed because she'd reply "yes" or "yay!" I suppose one of the reasons we would butt heads at times was not only because I was her firstborn but also because I was very headstrong and opinionated, just like she was. And controlling. There's no point denying it, since I have some distance from it now, and I can view it as the part of me that gets shit done. I don't hesitate when in a pinch. I act decisively. I choose swiftly, whether it ends up working out or not. I take the risk. I make the mistakes. And I'm willing to learn (more so now than when I was younger, of course). My mom was as pragmatic as they come. I am not as much. However, I'd follow her lead because I trusted her. For example, whenever she was feeling something happening in her body that was "off," I would ask her to "diagnose" herself first. When she had an issue with her kidneys after her big cancer surgery, she knew it was her kidneys before we confirmed it medically. She needed to have ureters (tubes) surgically placed so everything would "flow" properly. She knew it before anyone else. I was always amazed at how in tune she was with her body. And I am learning this for myself in large and small ways as I get older.

It is in these moments that I shared in my journal that I am now able to accept our relationship for all that it was and all that it was not. It was a payoff I wasn't thinking of at the time when we were in those cancer trenches together. I can see it clearly now and with a bittersweet joy that brings a smile and sometimes a tear.

After my mom died, one of my nephews chose to get a tattoo of his RahRah's first name, "Rosemary," on his rib cage. Because of our Arabic (actually, Chaldean) heritage (my mom was 100 percent Chaldean), my nephew did his research and found the characters in Arabic. I loved this idea so much that I copied it. My mom was not a fan of tattoos in the least. If she had known I was even considering having ink put on my skin, she would have objected while giving me that side eye, saying, "Lynnnnnnn!"

On the other hand, my mom also had enough of an ego that she would have loved the idea of her name being etched on my shoulder. I always feel like she is right here with me and will never really leave, so I know she'd approve of that as well.

Further Inquiry

You will, undoubtedly, come up with creative ways for you to express yourself while honoring your loved one. What other forms of expression can you think of? What have you done, heard of, or would like to try?

*"Self-care looks like
knowing what you need,
asking for what you need, and
expecting to receive
what you need.
Both from yourself and others."*

–@spiritdaughter, Instagram

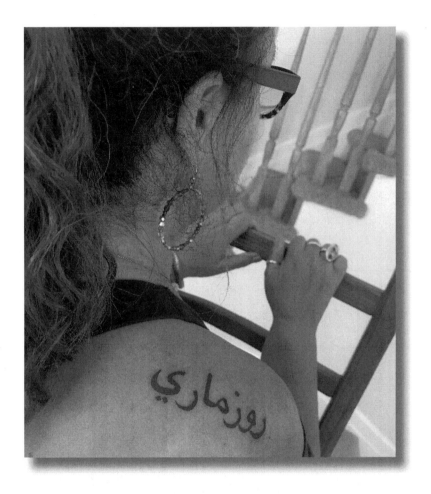

"Rosemary" in Arabic

LYNN ABATÉ-JOHNSON

This Is Real

Yesterday brought a cancer-journey milestone for RAH, and once again, just like when she got her diagnosis, she didn't even flinch. We were having a little hospital "beauty spa" moment while she was getting her blood transfusion in bed, complete with facial cleanser, warm washcloth, and a comb for her hair. She noticed that her hair was coming out a bit more than usual, so we concluded that the hair loss had indeed begun. We both just noticed it and smiled, then went on combing and tossing the hair in the rubbish bin. She wondered aloud if other hair (nostrils, eyebrows) would disappear, and we figured yes, it would. RAH is truly amazing. She seems prepared for anything and never complains in the process.

At times like this, I realized that I needed to suck it up and make the best of the new milestone. Her hair had started to fall out. We knew it was inevitable. My mom didn't let on that she was upset about it, even if she was. I followed her lead, and we chose to let it flow. Still, when something is inevitable, that doesn't mean we automatically have to be okay with it, or even embrace it. So many layers of life lessons came during this particular hospital stay. Embracing something that we don't like may make it more palatable, and still, it's difficult to do. Now that I have some distance from this formerly (in my mind) earth-shattering moment, I can remember how my mom faced it with such grace and her wonderful pragmatism. I need practice in this area, for sure.

Further Inquiry

How have you been able to manage hitting certain milestones in your journey? It may be helpful to express this in writing at some point.

"One of the hardest things is watching the world carry on while yours has crumbled."

–@thegriefspace_, Instagram

Is It True Now?

Standing at the hospital bathroom sink this morning, RAH was brushing her hair and pulling out a fair amount of it with each brush stroke.

Me: "See ya later, hair."

RAH: "After a while, alligator."

Our little mama exemplifies a positive outlook in all situations. Her oncologist told RAH it will be much better for her to be at home in her own environment than in the hospital, where she has so much artificial stuff going into her body, which she needed at the time, but now it's time to get back to her more natural environment.

While being released to finally go home was a big yay(!), it was also sometimes an "oh no!"

Are we ready? Are we organized? Can we take care of her at home without the extra medical staff buzzing around? I remember these questions running through my mind, and again, my sense of responsibility (and a bit of anxiety, of course) coming into play.

In these circumstances, I put one foot in front of the other and learned to navigate the unsteady and unpredictable circumstances the best way possible. So, yes, let's get her back to her own home, and her own comfy bed and other surroundings, and we'll take it from there, come what may.

I don't remember in all those years even getting so much as a cold or sniffle. And neither did my mom. Her oncologist once remarked that other than the cancer, she was as healthy as they come! I used to fear that she'd get pneumonia in the hospital during one of her stays, or bedsores from being at home in bed so much. I worried for nothing. And I've learned to normalize the worry, the anxiety, the conflict, and the not knowing. The ideas, opinions, assessments, and all my judgments came into play when I was thrust into this life-and-death challenge. I powered through. I made "it" work, whatever the "it" was at any given moment. That's what we do, right?

We take what's in front of us, and in knowing that it's not our time to fall apart, we plow ahead. And with every unnecessary worry that never turned out to be a bigger deal, like all the hospital visits that did not bring horrible additional issues, I learned to soothe myself in new ways I still use today.

"Is it true now?" Asking myself this question in the moment helped diffuse my worry. Judging the present experience against the past or in fear of the future outcome is a fruitless endeavor. It is only at this moment that we can develop more knowledge from the information at hand. We get to choose (and we always have a choice) when we consider a challenge. What do we believe in the current moment? I like to think I modeled some of my mom's pragmatic style in learning to assess where we were at a specific time. I developed a balanced approach so I didn't spin off the rails either way (imminent doom or denial).

Another way of reframing in any given circumstance centered around the word "balance." Balance is a word that is super subjective to the point of being meaningless for me. I think "balance" has become a buzzword, somewhat mythical. So, for us mortals dealing with such intense drama here on earth, I believe the best we can do is the best we can do, without being concerned about all that "normalcy" and "balance." What we feel in this moment is part of our own leadership and growth journeys as human beings holding so much love (and heaviness, at times).

Additionally, I've gradually cut out of my thinking and vocabulary the word *should*. There is really no such thing as should. When I was going through a divorce many lifetimes ago (first marriage), my counselor told me not to "should" on myself. I was constantly second-guessing and comparing myself to others, and it only led to more heartbreak and frustration. The more I reject **comparisons** and "shoulds" in my daily circumstances and choices, the more peace I cultivate in my soul. It's truly been a game changer in my life and in my business.

Further Inquiry

There is a lot to unpack here. "Is it true now?" If you wish, write down this question and tuck it away in your pocket as a reminder to stay in the moment and not let the "what if" fear get in the way. There's doing the best you can, while you can. And there is being aware of how often you "should" on yourself, or make comparisons. Which of these do you need right now? Take a moment and think it through. Apply it and see if it has an impact on your present state.

"People often think there is no way to heal from severe loss. I believe that is not true. You heal when you can remember those who have died with more love than pain, when you find a way to create meaning in your own life in a way that will honor theirs. It requires a decision and a desire to do this, but finding meaning is not extraordinary, it's ordinary. It happens all the time, all over the world."

–David Kessler, *Finding Meaning: The Sixth Stage of Grief*

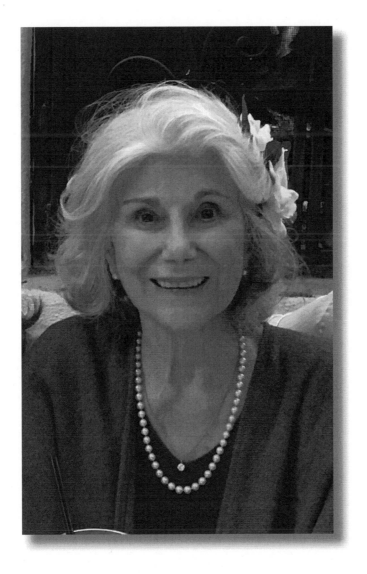

Eightieth birthday party: making that gardenia look more beautiful.

Surrender to Discomfort

Round three–hospital again. This morning, as Team RahRah tried to administer RAH's morning meds, antibiotics, etc., RAH vomited and couldn't even keep water down. Still extremely constipated and weak, in pain, and unable to get anything in that would help her, the call was made to get to the hospital and get some relief for her. What a trooper. Nicole spent the day getting her into the ED and admitted into a room. RAH is feeling a bit better. She has had some minor release of the constipation and has received IV antibiotics and blood thinner for the clot in her leg, and she is resting. She has been sleeping on and off all day. Her spirits are good overall. We hope that she continues to relax so that she'll feel much better tomorrow. At least she is in a place where she can be fed what she needs through the IV until her bowels return to normal. She is dealing with that, plus the abdominal infection, plus the blood clot. None of these is a small thing, but they're all manageable. We just aren't equipped to do it at home on our own, so RAH is doing round three at the hospital. She'll be okay, we just need to make sure she gets over this hump so her body functions normally, allowing her to move around, eat, drink, heal.

Around the time my mom started her chemotherapy treatments, she started whispering. And even when she spoke a little more than a whisper, her voice was hoarse. It freaked me out. A friend stopped by to visit her.

"She is in a state of grace," the friend said. I will always remember that moment. A "state of grace?" What the F is that? Ugh. No! I don't like it. That's not *my mom*!

What does that even mean? "State of grace." I looked it up, years later, and aside from the religious interpretation, I can see in hindsight that my mom was in a state of surrender, relinquishing control, quieting her mind, body, and spirit. This was very uncomfortable for me to witness as her daughter. She never whispered. She would never in her life relinquish control. She was a fighter! She could conquer any monster, any adversary, with her sheer will. That didn't work so well in the case of her cancer journey. She did try to fight many times though.

I needed help understanding the fact that my mom's personality seemed to be changing. She was fighting off the dis-ease in her body. She whispered, and it made me uncomfortable, but that was my own shit to work out, not a flaw in her personality or some perceived weirdness. I can see now that it was a natural facet of my mom's unique journey through the very darkest of times, as there was a war happening between the dis-ease and the way her brain, body, and soul navigated it all.

It is a normal course in the journey for a loved one's behavior (and our own, for that matter) to become unrecognizable and far from the way things were before the diagnosis. And once again, leaving "should" (and comparisons) out of the equation helps here. Where there was once power and control, there is now surrender and perceived weakness. It's far from a weakness, however, and the shift in our mindsets when things like this come up to challenge our thinking are worth examining and grappling with.

Further Inquiry

What beliefs have you noticed thus far in your caregiving journey that you could let go of? Are there things you're holding on to about your loved one that you could release (even if it's temporary) in order to give your loved one space? I have found, through my own distance and introspection, that relinquishing control and "shoulds" have had an immeasurable effect on me, and I believe that a practice of letting go will benefit you as well once the uncomfortable becomes comfortable, or at least accepted as "what is" for the moment at any given point in your journey with your loved one(s).

"There are stars whose radiance is visible on Earth though they have long been extinct.
There are people whose brilliance continues to light the world even though they are no longer among the living.
These lights are particularly bright when the night is dark. They light the way for humankind."

–Hannah Senesh, Instagram

Trust

Today is my birthday. The day my mom gave birth to me. It's amazing to think about where my mom was a year ago today, still at "Happy Acres," the local Skilled Nursing Facility, weighing all of 79 lbs and just starting to grow her hair back after the longest summer of our lives. In hindsight, I can say it was worth it. Because today, I have been reflecting about how grateful I am to still have my mom to wish a happy "birth day" to (since she birthed me, it's a celebration for her as well!). RAH is continuing her healing journey, becoming more and more fierce about gaining her strength and regularity back. Yes, there is still plenty of time on the "throne!" ha ha ha

She goes to the local farmers' markets at least once a week. She's juicing often, which makes a huge difference for ALL of us who are also drinking the stuff. She's on EVERYONE's case about being tested for the same BRCA 2 5804 deleterious mutation that she has. She's becoming a regular Sherlock Holmes on behalf of all of us in the family to be sure that our children and their children know ahead of time if they have to deal with the potential hazards of having the mutated gene. RAH is making her own doctor and therapy appointments and is getting HERSELF UP in the mornings, getting dressed, and getting out the door and off for activities; other days, she has time "off" (as she calls it), when she can just relax and enjoy one of her good trashy novels. It's such a joy to see my mom enjoying her life, her children, and her grandchildren. She is getting in "our business," caring about how we are doing, soothing furrowed brows, and taxing our patience again (at times) with her endless wisdom and lessons.

I will say that my mom did, indeed, appear to live a life with no regrets. She was full of joy during times when she was on an upswing during her journey. And that's enough for me. I'm learning to trust more and more with each passing year. For me, this is a part of **practicing something that I know many caregivers are in the throes of: trusting.** Since my mom died, I realized there was trust missing. Trusting myself and my instincts. Trusting my mom and her instincts. Back then, I thought I trusted (intellectually); however, I've since realized that I need to listen to myself more deeply—to my body, heart, soul—and a bit less to my head. Often, getting out of my head (and into a place of trust) is as simple as pausing and breathing deeply. I have tried many modalities to get in touch with other parts of me when I'm getting too "heady." As my mom would have said, "I'm a tough nut to crack in that area." I used to hold tightly to my thoughts, to a fault, rather than tap into my feelings and my body. Recently, I've been practicing something called "square breathing technique," and for me, it helps. From there, I can tap into my heart, soul, and spirit, all of which hold all the wisdom I need. Giving my thoughts a break has been useful over these transformational years. Knowing how to navigate all these centers of "knowingness" has held keys that unlock places I never thought about before. In fact, it's what has me here, writing about my continuing journey.

I used to think during those years when my mom was on the down part of the roller coaster, with her cancer and treatment slowly killing her, that she had lost her instincts to "mother" us. To me, her "mothering us" looked like curiosity (about us and our lives, including her grandchildren's) and in the way she was always teaching us. She stopped asking us about ourselves, our lives, and the kids, and she stopped instructing us on the normal everyday things we were used to. She even stopped telling us to take off our shoes at the door and to wash our hands (gasp!). I wondered whether she cared about us anymore.

Months passed in that first year without the typical small talk or updates about what we were up to. She often seemed to be focused on "nothingness." She seemed to be in such a mindless fog at times. I learned later that it had nothing to do with her loving or caring about us. It had everything to do with her energy, mainly conserving it, whether she was aware of that on the surface or not. It was literally impossible for her to muster those teaching moments. It was her turn to be cared for and loved. That much she knew, instinctively. To me, it looked like indifference. How wrong I was!

So, in modeling this new behavior, she actually *did* teach me about life and dying. Once again, I went from making it all about me to finding ways to understand my mother's capacity to love while fighting for her life in ways neither of us could have prepared for. This was so different in my experience as her daughter. And I am grateful for it, in hindsight.

Further Inquiry

What previous characteristics of your loved one are missing at this moment? Life has a way of changing us as we move through our challenges. How do you get "out of your head" and tap into your heart when faced with uncomfortable realizations?

"Go and love someone exactly as they are.
And then watch how quickly they
transform
into the greatest, truest,
version of themselves.
When one feels seen and
appreciated in their own
essence, one is instantly
empowered."

–Wes Angelozzi

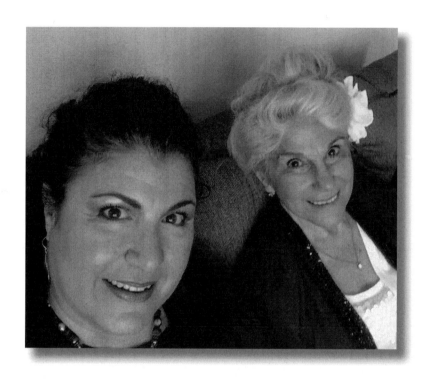

Hanging out together, trusting all is well.

There's a Reason—Or Is There?

It's been a while since my last update on RAH and, as usual, no news is good news, at least in this case. RAH is being watched like baby birds are watched by their parents. She has a capable and loyal team of doctors, as well as other health practitioners, who are keeping a close eye on her while she continues to regain strength, stamina, muscle tone (yep!), and endurance. She is still going to yoga class two to three times a week, and she is working out at a local gym with a personal trainer who continually challenges her to grow in her strength. It has been a real treat to watch as she progresses. She's also getting three massages each week and lymphatic treatments / physical therapy to help her lymphatic system since so many of her lymph nodes were removed in 2011. Her surgeon, her oncologist, and her survival specialist (expert in BRCA2 genetics) are just a few of the doctors who are monitoring her. Right now, RAH is enjoying reading

a book by Dr. Wayne Dyer on visualization. She typ-
ically reads fiction, but now she's reading a self-help
book! We're happy as long as she's reading because
it's a good sign, so we'll take it. By next month, hope-
fully, RAH will be going on her next trip, or at least
planning it. We are SO fortunate. We don't take it
lightly that RAH is thriving after such a potentially
devastating bout with cancer. And this realization
leaves us grateful beyond words. We visualize health
and happiness for each of you, as we are doing for
RAH, so that we can continue to enjoy the lives we've
been given here on the planet together. Thank you for
your love and constant caring.

I remember feeling afraid to hope, especially when she was on an upswing. I learned that my fears and anxieties were made up because my emotions spun sometimes. I navigated them the best I could, and mainly in silence. I knew in my mind and heart that this was all part of the deal.

My youngest sister used to say that she thought the reason our mama got sick was to teach us about that journey, with all its nuances, including the horror and beauty of it. I believe this too. It makes sense to me, and especially when we need it to make sense. That was a rational anchor for us as we rode the cancer roller coaster together.

I learned (and I'm still learning) to **navigate the hurt, anger, sadness, and feelings of being abandoned and neglected.** Seeing someone who birthed and raised me be so graceful and strong in the face of terrifying odds was sobering, to say the least. And, at the same time, I am open and curious to this day about how we, as humans, can navigate the complexity of exactly this: being human.

Further Inquiry

How have you been doing in navigating the complexities of your unique journey? Write down those things so you can refer back to them at a later date. You are going to amaze yourself, I bet!

"There is no way to be a perfect mother and a million ways to be a good one."

–Jill Churchill

Getting a Grip

RAH has been doing really well since she returned from a trip to Florida. In fact, I haven't heard her so excited about how great she's feeling. She has a cheery disposition, and when I acknowledge that, she often says something like "I'm feeling so great!" or "Everything is working in my body—I think it's all the greens!" She's sleeping well, eating well, her weight is steady (they say that lots of living foods will regulate your weight to a healthy normal for each individual) . . . all is well! It is music to our ears and a feast for our eyes to see RAH smiling, glowing, and thriving! If you had seen her in 2011, you might have thought this was NEVER going to happen, especially after such a dismal diagnosis and horrific surgery and treatment/ aftermath. RAH always says, "I'll tell you when to worry." Even through the fog of all the drugs she has to take, she knows more than any of us.

When we got news that my mom's metabolic panel came back with some new "activity" and a dear family member suggested a place in Florida where she could go live for three weeks to strengthen her system with living foods, we made it happen. And as you can see from this journal entry, it was a good call.

We figured that even though my mom hesitated to spend her money on this adventure, it would at least be a break for her to see if three weeks on greens and other living foods would help her tolerate the new chemo regimen we knew was inevitable. And it seemed to do just that.

However, prior to that, there was a very dark time when she was so medically unstable that we weren't equipped at home for the level of care she needed. I remember driving around with Corey between Napa and Sonoma visiting Skilled Nursing Facilities, and at one of them, I came back to the car in tears because it was so disgusting and smelled so gross when I walked through the front door. I could not and would not subject my mom to that type of place. So, I needed to pull myself together and find something suitable for her acute care needs. We finally settled for the "lesser of evils," and although we weren't able to spend the nights there with her, we were never far away. We arranged scheduled visits with local friends who smuggled treats into her room for her and hung out with her in between the times we were there, so she was never alone for too long during the daytime hours. I nicknamed the place "Happy Acres" because there was nothing "happy" about it. I hated that she had to be there, and yet we didn't have a choice. It was the responsible thing to do. Temporarily.

And still, I grappled with feelings of anger and resentment that I could not do everything for her. I had to find ways to rationalize what was not mine to carry. In the years since my mom's death, I've developed a new mantra that helps me embrace those emotions I used to think were selfish and unnecessary. Hint: They are all necessary, and now, welcome.

My mantra today: "Is this mine to carry?"

My mom didn't need me hovering over her. In fact, it was detrimental at times for her and our relationship. It became clear to me after most of that first year passed that my mom often rallied and did better when I wasn't hovering over her. I needed to force myself to stay away and let others fill in. I was frequently too involved to the point where it wasn't good for her or for me to be there in person. So I did my best to check in from a distance and manage my own inner conflict and anxiety about leaving control to others in our circle. I remember saying to my mom that it was a good thing she had five kids!

When I couldn't be with my mom, I cried at home. You keep your shit together and do what is necessary to be of service out of love for your family member or friend and then allow yourself those moments to let it all out.

The tears, the rage, the loneliness, the despair—they all needed to vent out of me like a pressure cooker, and each unique human might process what I experienced differently. It's such an individual and personal thing, and it was how I grieved. I was staying with my mom on most weekdays because my husband was traveling for work, and so when he'd come home on the weekends, I'd go home to be with him. That's when I'd let my emotions flow. What I know for sure is that this process needs to happen in some healthy way, shape, or form.

To my surprise and delight, I have learned that caregivers have organized all over the world.

I hadn't realized this until I became a caregiver myself. In many local areas, in-person and online resources are available for support, thus allowing caregivers the foundation of self-care they need on their personal journey.

I remember seeing things like "Yoga for Caregivers" and other cool activities that surfaced after my mom died. A good friend of mine leads meditations and workshops for mindful caregiving. Pretty powerful, magical, valuable stuff. Please see the Resources section in the back of the book for people and ideas you can start with. Additionally, an online search for local resources will come in handy for you. How reassuring to know we're not alone and that there are people trained to support us through some of the most uncertain times in our lives.

Further Inquiry

Where is your safe spot to vent? The car? The laundry room? When everyone finally leaves the house? Wherever it is, protect that space and use it as frequently as you need to. It's better to let it all out than to bottle it up inside. Easier said than done, I understand.

"To care for those who cared for us is one of the highest honors."

–Peggi Speers and Tia Walker, *The Inspired Caregiver: Finding Joy While Caring for Those You Love*

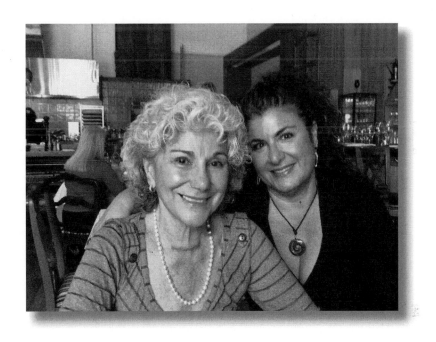

Evenings out together.

We'll Take It!

RAH *went in a bit early for her monthly check-in with her oncologist. He told her that she was perfectly healthy and that all her blood results were great except for the CA125 (which is in a steady climb). That's the tumor marker for ovarian cancer. The verdict is that she's starting chemotherapy again this Friday! I'll be with her all day at the hospital. She said she could go on her own, but you know that doesn't fly with me in this case.*

She's been having some days when she's tired and without her usual stamina. Like I said to her yesterday, for anyone else it would seem like "normal" stamina, but when she slows down and is tired during the day, we know that's a symptom.

RAH is very confident (and thus, so are we) that she'll get the chemo four to six times (cycles), then be done with it again (for a while, at least). She'll then heal from the aftereffects in time to have more fun in her retirement. She's planning a couple trips. So this firecracker that is our RahRah is not done yet by ANY means. Just a little bump and we'll be sticking closer to her than ever to shore her up in any way we can.

Before, during, and after those cancer years with my mom, you could often hear us use the expression "we'll take it." When we were in the thick of it and there were so many seemingly minor wins (and some big ones as well), every bit of good news we received was met with "we'll take it," usually initiated by my mom. It was yet another coping mechanism for us, and it worked well. We still say it today. We also express gratitude and celebration of our wins with "Very good! Very good! Yayyyyyy!" (Those of you who have experienced "laughter yoga" will know exactly what I'm referring to!)

I had taken laughter yoga classes prior to my mom's diagnosis. My youngest sister, Nicole, also took a bunch of classes with me, as did my mom. That saying morphed into a way of coping with whatever little good news we heard along the journey. CA-125 number went down? Meds or cannabis doing the job it's supposed to? "We'll take it!" and then "Very good! Very good! Yayyyyyy!" We'd always clap our hands and then hold our arms up in a V while saying yay! We'd all join in and giggle, including anyone who happened to be in the room at the time.

Nicole, a mom of three herself, coached me to "look at the whole picture" rather than one moment of one day when I panicked because something was "wrong" or "off," or anytime we'd have to make a run to the hospital emergency departments. It took years for me to adjust to this "big picture" thinking, and it was painful as hell. I look back on it now and chalk it up to my own growing pains as a human and as a daughter who was caught off guard. The lessons continue for me, even without my mom right here by my side. She's still (and forever) teaching me. And when Nicole can sense, even from a long distance, that I'm panicking, she texts me these words: "Stop freaking out."

"We'll take it" was always an acknowledgment that while we cannot control every outcome directly, we can view even the smallest things as a positive move toward a healthy outcome, or at least one that wasn't going to make the situation worse. Baby steps, small victories—we grasped *every single one*. And we celebrated in all these ways and more.

Further Inquiry

What are you grateful for at this moment? Gratitude (often in the form of "we'll take it") usually shifts my perspective in all the best ways.

"Nature does not hurry, yet everything is accomplished."

–Lao Tzu

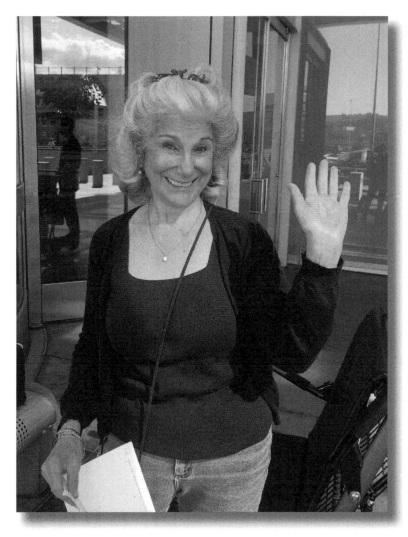

"See you later, alligator"/airport drop-off.

Six Years In

It's been six years since RAH's body started puffing up like a blowfish and she couldn't keep up at our morning exercise classes. We got a diagnosis within a week—ovarian cancer, stage IIIC (I've since nicknamed it "the gift that keeps on giving"). It's been a very full six years for RAH. We are super fortunate for every day we've enjoyed her being up and at 'em, bossing us all around, being larger than life and still in charge, even through some fairly dicey downturns. Although the last procedure (pleurocentesis) took a lot out of her, and the chemotherapy dosing has been a challenge, RAH's been staying pretty much ahead of the cancer cells that have been lurking and reoccurring in her system off and on all these years.

Last week's check-in with her oncologist brought us news that we didn't like. RAH's tumor marker came in very high. It really jumped up high in a short time. RAH wrote about this in a message to her siblings and children: "All I could think was 'wow.'"

It sucked. Almost every bit of every circumstance during those years sucked. And also, it didn't completely suck. I've learned to appreciate what happens in our bodies, minds, souls, spirits, and nervous systems when cancer happens. I've also been learning and continuously practicing curiosity as a way of being, especially when I think I have things figured out.

Rather than seeing contradictions, I am now practicing ways to view paradox, which has lightened up my view of life's conditions and circumstances. I never understood the concept of paradox as well as I have these past few years, especially since my mom died. Because of my mom's encouragement, her voice in my head, I've been brought to a place where I've learned the following: I used to think of contradiction as being a weakness; now I see it as an opportunity to explore life as a paradox. That's a broad inquiry, I know—a big distinction. Through my own thoughts and tapping into my intuition when I was considering making a career move after my mom's death, I sensed my mom "guide" me to apply for the position I currently hold with the leadership development and professional coach training company, Co-Active Training Institute—CTI. I continue to learn about perspective as well! Paradox and perspective have been game-changers for my mindset and mental agility.

Learning to take a special delight in differences never occurred to me. In fact, back when Corey and I were struggling in our marriage (What did we know? We were young!), we would lament about the differences between us. What a soul-satisfying freedom it has become to recognize that yes, we are very different in many ways, and wow, what a gift that is for our relationship and the growth we can tap in to as individuals. So, I think of my mom with so much gratitude for helping guide me and for believing in me, even after she left her physical body. She gave me the gifts of learning more about myself and my outlook on things that I *thought* I knew so well. And the lessons keep coming.

Further Inquiry

When the news about your loved one is bad, what kinds of conversations do you have with yourself and others? Once time passes, after the initial shock subsides, what else is revealed in your personal journey?

"... humanity will reach maturity and wisdom on the day that it begins not just to tolerate but take a special delight in differences ..."

–Gene Roddenberry

Being a Bad Daughter

Good news: *RAH is gaining weight. Gaining strength. Weaning off most chemical medications. For example, even with RAH being full of, well, "full of it," she will eat a full meal and then ask what is for snack right afterward! Since RAH has left "Happy Acres" (the Skilled Nursing Facility), no one has had to sleep over with her. She has been coherent and participatory in a very strong way, both emotionally and physically. Even her voice is really strong! RAH has a great attitude most of the time.*

Bad news: *RAH has fluid retention again. It seems like more this time around, but is it because the loculations (scar tissue) have broken up and it has spread more? This could be a good and a bad thing—good that scar tissue is broken up, but bad that there is more fluid. RAH's system is still confused. One minute she is constipated and the next minute she has diarrhea. Maybe the reduction of medications will help work* *this out. RAH feels stuffed and has challenges moving with so much fluid. This is the most we have seen in a while, so it is a bit worrisome.*

Was I a bad daughter? I met with a good friend of thirty-plus years recently, and we talked about caring for our moms as they age while also being caregivers for various other loved ones in our lives. We are part of what is sometimes referred to as the "sandwich generation." Our lives are "sandwiched" between our elderly family members and our children (and often grandchildren). I can relate so well to what many of my friends and acquaintances feel and internalize about themselves and their very identities. It's deeply personal stuff, the conversations we've had about this. How many times did I think to myself that I was being a "bad daughter" or a "bitch" during the years my mom was fighting cancer? Too many to count.

I remember times when my mom (feeling well and energetic enough to go out to eat, shop, have some fun) asked me to accompany her and I'd feel terrible saying no. I never wanted to say no to my mom because I knew that 1) being with her was a way to honor and enjoy her, and 2) I could feel her time on the planet fading away, so I always sensed a ticking clock. I remember saying to my mom on such an occasion, "I feel like I'm being a bad daughter, Mom, but I cannot take time away from work."

I used to have the same experience in my body. I felt like I was being a bad daughter when out of pure love (and if I'm being truthful, often fear mixed with desperation to help "save" my mom), I'd badger her (yes, it's a strong word and that's exactly how it felt at times . . . to her and to me listening in):

"Please drink your water, Mom." (She hated drinking water, and it filled up her tiny little tummy. Often, it was either that or nourishing food for her to choose between.)

"Mom, remember that cancer loves sugar. Please eat something else that helps your body fight."

(My mom was addicted to sugar, as was I. Her doctors said to let her eat and drink whatever she wanted. Those were the times I wanted to "fight" them.)

Her surgeon, after her stay at the hospital after her original surgery, stopped in to say goodbye as we were heading home, finally. Prior to my mom's diagnosis, I learned about alkalinity in the body and its benefits. I asked the doctor what he thought about doing whatever we could to keep her body in balance with alkalinity as a cornerstone. He said that he thought it was bullshit, but we could do what we want. (I will never forget it, and that was February 2011.)

Fast-forward a few years later. I took my mom to this same surgeon to have her port removed from her shoulder. She was feeling really well, like she had beaten the cancer, so she wanted that chemo port removed. We were catching up on life in general, and the surgeon said that he'd recently been in Europe, spent time at a cooking school of some sort, and that he was writing a cancer-fighting cookbook. It was vegetarian! My mom and I, remembering how he dismissed our alkalinity question years prior, gave each other a "knowing" look and softly smiled without saying anything.

Among the many threads woven into the tapestry of our cancer journey together, nutrition was a big deal, and often, with conflicting advice coming at us, a bone of contention. My mom would sometimes say "stop bugging me," or she'd have friends who visited (often helping us care for her) sneak in "contraband" in the form of sweets and snacks. It took me years to finally calm myself down and learn to keep my mouth shut in the face of her choices and cravings (and a shrink would have a field day with this, knowing these were all reflections of the way I neglected my own health and nutrition for many years, to my detriment).

Further Inquiry

What have you noticed rearing up between you and your loved one(s) that has you questioning yourself? I have found that writing these down and talking to a trusted confidant really helps.

"You are not a bad caregiver if you:
Don't enjoy caregiving.
Do things your loved one doesn't
want you to do.
Hire a caregiver to help so you can
get a break.
Get grossed out by aspects of
caregiving.
Put your loved one in a care facility.
Look forward to the caregiving
journey ending.
Daydream about not doing
anything.
Want to be alone from time to time.
Sleep in a different room than your
loved one."

–@dementia_careblazers, Instagram

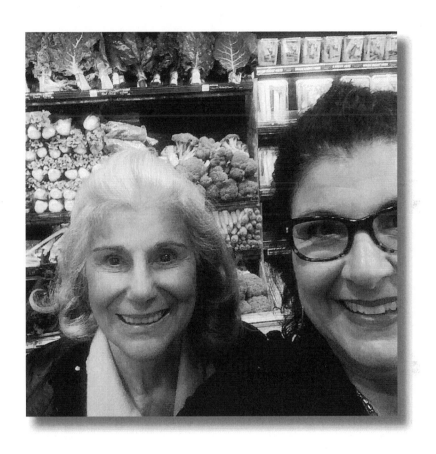

I loved running into her in the produce aisles.

Ask for Support

RAH and I have had some conversations lately about the time since her diagnosis, death, life, and all the experiences we have faced. She doesn't remember a LOT, especially during all the months of being medicated for pain, in and out of emergency rooms, hospitals stays, and "Happy Acres." She is really sharp, she just doesn't relate to certain things. For example, when her neighbor reminded her of all the vomiting, RAH said it was because of swallowing pills. She doesn't realize that the chemo really did a number on her, along with the cancer, so she still doesn't believe the chemo made her throw up. Swallowing all those pills was just a catalyst at times, along with eating certain foods that triggered her cough/ allergy spasms. Hopefully, that's all behind RAH, and the upswing in her health will continue.

Get additional support in any way possible. I remember coming on strong once or twice, letting my mom know I was exhausted. And in my more "drama queen" moments, I'd say, "Your cancer is killing me, Mom." That's when I got the true meaning of what others before me had written about, saying that cancer is a family dis-ease. Everyone is affected. So true for me. I'm grateful that my mom didn't feel an ounce of guilt. Between forgetting and being pragmatic, she could see how intense the experience was for her children and grandchildren. She was able to detach from guilt and still relate to my expressions of exhaustion. She modeled being okay with my "stuff" in the moment rather than taking it on. She had enough to deal with, on all levels, and yet I felt completely free to express my own emotions to her. I remember a good friend of ours who helped care for her telling me that my mom was worried about me. So she heard me, and she saw me.

Still, when you are a caregiver, the energetic drain is present, or it can be, if you don't figure out healthy ways to navigate around all that and take breaks to truly recharge. I was never able to fully recharge.

Although I know I did a *pretty good* job with what I had to deal with in front of me, moment to moment, the essence of my energetic nervous system was that this whole experience was really about *me* and how I was facing life without my mom. I allowed myself to go through most of that first year having what I called a "pity party" for myself in facing the very real possibility that my mom was going to "get dead" from cancer.

My visiting aunts noticed my anxiety was robbing me of sleep. They recommended I try just a tiny dose of Ativan. I had never considered using anything to help me with my anxiety and sleeplessness, yet I did try the lowest dose once a day for a bit. It helped, but then I started to feel like I needed to up the dose, so I stopped taking it. I didn't want to risk getting addicted to any sort of drug. Instead, I went to a healer I'd heard about and ended up replacing the Ativan with herbs (like Tulsi/Holy Basil) to help calm my nervous system.

To this day, I still use herbs to help calm my very active brain at night.

Further Inquiry

What kinds of remedies work (or worked) well for you?
How do you practice self-care in the toughest moments?

"Our deepest fear is not that we are inadequate. Our deepest fear is that we are powerful beyond measure. It is our light, not our darkness that most frightens us. We ask ourselves, who am I to be brilliant, gorgeous, talented and fabulous? Actually, who are you not to be? You are a child of God. Your playing small doesn't serve the world. There's nothing enlightened about shrinking so that other people won't feel insecure around you. We were born to make manifest the glory of God that is within us. It's not just in some of us; it's in everyone. And as we let our own light shine, we unconsciously give other people permission to do the same. As we are liberated from our own fear, our presence automatically liberates others."

–Marianne Williamson, *A Return to Love: Reflections on the Principles of "A Course in Miracles"*

"Eat the Fish, Bitch!"

RAH had another restful night of sleep. Yesterday, when she was getting up from an afternoon nap, she remarked how much easier it is to get around without worrying about her bladder or bowel issues and the accompanying Foley or self-catheter system. That, in itself, is a big deal and a milestone. And without the catheter, RAH has a better chance of warding off any further urinary tract or yeast infections. It seems the injection last week did the trick to help with RAH's blood levels. So far, no recent trips to the hospital, and RAH's weight is at 95, same as last week (but at least not lower). Eating and drinking enough to not only sustain herself but also try to pack on more energy in the form of calories is proving to be quite a challenge for RAH, so we are really trying to help her stay on top of it, along with managing her tummy pain, which is not nearly as severe this week as it had been.

In the 2013 film featuring Julia Roberts as the daughter and Meryl Streep as the mom with cancer, *August: Osage County*, there is a scene where Julia's character is sitting at the dinner table with her mom and the rest of the family. The mom is not eating much. The daughter starts in on her mother:

"Eat the fish. Eat the fish. Eat the fish." Finally, she screams, "Eat the fish, bitch!"

I remember that scene so vividly; it's as if it happened at my mom's dinner table. It never did, but it felt like it very well could have. I laughed and cried simultaneously watching this scene in the film. I remember relaying my experience of it to my mom later when she was feeling healthy and more like herself. I confessed to her that I felt the same way sometimes, mostly out of frustration and in wanting my mom to be able to eat and enjoy her food and the nourishment it could bring her, while also being so agitated that we found ourselves in this ridiculous cancer situation. Ugh! I wanted my mom to "eat the fish!" for herself and for me.

Granted, my frustration and desperation at the time were warranted. My normally fit, healthy mom was wasting away. My fear of her dying from starvation was real and visceral (I can actually still feel it in the pit of my stomach). I used to "joke" with my mom, saying stuff like "imagine you, the healthiest, most food-loving person I have ever known, dying not of cancer but of starvation." I couldn't fathom it. And so I tried to control it, and her behavior. The truth is, at the time, I was desperate to control my mom's food intake for sheer survival. I realized later that no matter how much love, effort, pleas, or tears I devoted, I couldn't get a handle on my own relationship with food, let alone help my mom with hers. It was also two very different scenarios. My mom physically could not eat at the time until she made it through some of her health milestones (which she eventually did, reversing her cachexia).

When my friends who are also caregivers for their moms tell me they feel like "bad daughters" or guilty for trying to help their moms take care of themselves, I get it. I lived it. When my mom would tell me to stop nagging at her, it was easy for me to turn it around on her as well. I'd tell her, "I learned how to care for you *from* you, Mom. In fact, if this situation were reversed, and I was the one with cancer, you would be relentless in your pursuit of the best nutrition and care possible for me. I nag you out of love, and I don't know how else to *be with* this."

She truly got it. She understood me because I was her in so many ways. In the same way as my mom was, I am capable, trustworthy, loyal, intelligent, and passionate. Mom loved and fought to stay on earth for me (and, of course, the rest of her family). I often had the feeling that many of the things I said out loud to her she already knew.

I wish I could tell my younger, scared-shitless-daughter-self to take care of herself. To do one thing each day that serves her highest good—her physical, spiritual, and emotional health. I'd tell her that one thing for her does not take anything away from her sick mama. One thing.

Small moments.

Tiny wins in the midst of the battle.

During those cancer years, I loaded 53 lbs of weight back onto my body after dieting the year prior to her diagnosis. And in the month leading up to her death, I packed on another 10 lbs, built almost solely on sugary coffee drinks. All the sugar fed my craving for a life with my healthy little mama on top of her game again.

Ironically, I used to think that the "weight" (not only physical weight, but also the "weight of the world") I carried out of neglect for my own needs was somehow helpful in service of my mom and others. Part of the irony was that this "weight" was extremely painful for my mom to see. She hated that I was overweight because she knew I was unhealthy, and she couldn't bear the thought of me dying from obesity in the same way one of her favorite aunts did. My mom let her emotions show sparingly. I rarely saw her cry. And yet when she told me the story of her obese aunt dying, she cried. And that's when I realized she was fearful of the same thing happening to me. The final irony in all this is that it wasn't until my mom left the planet that I started taking better care of my health.

My mom was also very savvy about finances. She was always trying to teach us to be fiscally responsible. "Have a cushion," she'd say. "Work hard, be productive, contribute to society and your community, earn money so you never have to depend on anyone else to care for you." She modeled this throughout her life.

The two main issues my mom had with me and how I lived *my* life were my physical and financial health, and it wasn't until she made her departure that I was able to grasp the importance of both. So today, I stand in a position of growth and self-care that I know she's proud to see from her perch on my shoulder.

Further Inquiry

If you could have a conversation with your younger self and your future self, what would you say to reassure them?

"Our relationships are reflections of the one we have with ourselves."

–@iyanlavanzant, Instagram

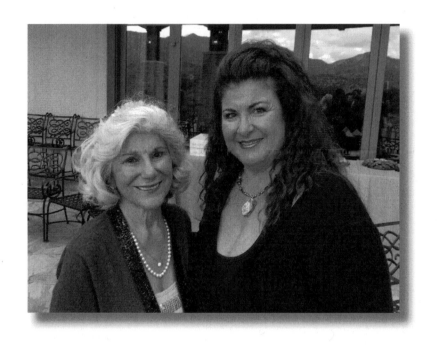

She starved. I ate for both of us.

Thanksgiving and Anticipatory Grief

RAH's first Thanksgiving Day while undergoing chemo-therapy finds her feeling better except for that pesky stomach business. She still has a tough time with almost constant abdominal pain. We'll gather for a modest Thanksgiving lunch at Nicole's today. RAH thought it would be nice to only prepare a few things our-selves, so she is doing the candied yams (one of her faves), Nicole is doing a kale salad, and I am doing a romaine salad and fresh (raw) cranberry/orange relish (it's amazing, if I do say so myself). In addition, RAH had a "field trip" to the grocer earlier this week where she taste-tested their Thanksgiving offerings. She ordered mashed potatoes, gravy, green beans, a turkey, and a pumpkin pie. She also picked up a can of whipped cream. We will heat up the pre-ordered food and enjoy it together with what we each prepare.

The food, and especially the gathering of her "crew" around the table, was one of my mom's favorite acts of love—feeding us and everyone eating together. Like me, one of her love-languages was feeding people. The holidays were a very big deal to my mom. She enjoyed cooking and eating food, and she enjoyed eating out too, like I did. She was super picky about ingredients when she shopped. She liked crisp, green, crunchy romaine lettuce leaves. My mom was the salad queen. I also became a salad queen, and to this day, when invited to a potluck, I'm assigned the salad. I wouldn't have it any other way because I get to buy fresh, organic produce, clean it and chop it, and make a masterpiece salad that everyone gobbles up. And I always make my own fresh salad dressing.

I have a theory that the reason my mom didn't get diagnosed with cancer until she was seventy-three, even while carrying the BRCA 2 genetic mutation, was because she was so healthy. She never carried extra weight on her body, never smoked, rarely drank, had an amazing constitution, and she slept well every night. She defied the statistics for others who carry that genetic mutation, and she outlived the statistics once she was diagnosed.

My mom's cancer journey taught me about how our bodies fight for us. Without getting into any medical or scientific jargon, here's what I learned during and after the cancer years: Inflammation and inflammatory dis-ease is prevalent. And, at times, invisible. Our bodies become inflamed with dis-ease. It's a protective mechanism, in a way. I had no clue about it before my mom had cancer. And even in the years since she died, I've been learning more about how it manifests in my own body. I never realized that things like arthritis, asthma, cancer, type 2 diabetes, fatty liver disease, auto-immune disorders, and even depression are linked to inflammation.

The good news is that inflammation is often completely reversible. The even better news is that food and nutrition can be the very medicine we might need, plus other overlooked things like sleep, hydration, and practices that make sense for each individual (like reading, music, mindfulness, hormone-balancing care, meditations, fresh air, etc.). The solutions are as varied as we are. Every *body* is different and yet there is much we have in common in terms of ways to come into better balance.

While I hesitate to give specific advice to anyone, I am happy to share what's worked for me over the years. I've developed some nonnegotiable regular practices, and I am always looking for new things to experience.

In terms of how I care for my whole self (body, mind, spirit), I love being outdoors, going for walks, staring at the Pacific Ocean while breathing deeply, riding my bicycle, roller-skating, belly dancing, and doing Pilates and other simple, functional movement practices. And I protect my sleep, fiercely.

Nutritionally, I have adopted, thanks to my dear friend, chef Bridget Foliaki-Davis, a gut-healthy lifestyle, which I practice daily. No more DIEting. I used to DIE-it. Now I LIVE-it, through eating healthy meals and drinking plenty of water. Fortunately, Bridget's meal plans are organized and ready for me to do the fun part—shop for fresh ingredients and get into my kitchen. I've always loved to cook. My mom was a fantastic cook, especially when we were younger, and she had seven mouths to feed on a very tight budget. Like my mom, feeding people is one of my love-languages, so when I discovered Bridget, her cookbooks and online meal plans, I uncovered a new way of life that benefits Corey and me in ways we never imagined possible. I sometimes wish my mom were still here to experience this food-love with me. Talk about anti-inflammatory!

As much as I loved the big gatherings with every family member plus guests (which added up to a giant crowd!), I have now created a different perspective. It is taking some practice on my part (and Corey's too). Each time a holiday approaches, and especially if it was a favorite of my mom's, I encourage my family and friends to be relaxed about gathering. Instead of making it all about the food/meal planning, which I still like to do, I focus on ease, fun, flow, love, and alignment, rather than the hustle and bustle and stress and strain on the few who are doing the prepping, hosting, cooking, and cleaning. Sorry, Mom. I can't do it the way we used to when you were alive. More guilt? Being a bad daughter again? Nope. It's me claiming my voice and prioritizing my physical and mental health in these matters.

When my mom was still at our holiday tables, I remember having anticipatory grief. I would envision every family gathering as our possible final one with her. I envisioned the next holiday being without her at the table, bustling in the kitchen, standing at the sink doing the cleanup, and working her tail off to serve us all when she was feeling strong.

I (and here's more normalization of my guilt complex) actually relished those years of holiday times when she was too weak or sick to fully participate, so we were able to cook for her and serve her. She directed from her seat, of course, still powerful and in charge but in a much different way. She was less preoccupied by the food; she learned to relinquish control, to slow down, and to let others be of service to her while she observed her family gathered around her.

Further Inquiry

How can you find ways to celebrate milestones in even more healthy ways for you and your loved ones? What kinds of inflammatory conditions have you noticed along your journey?

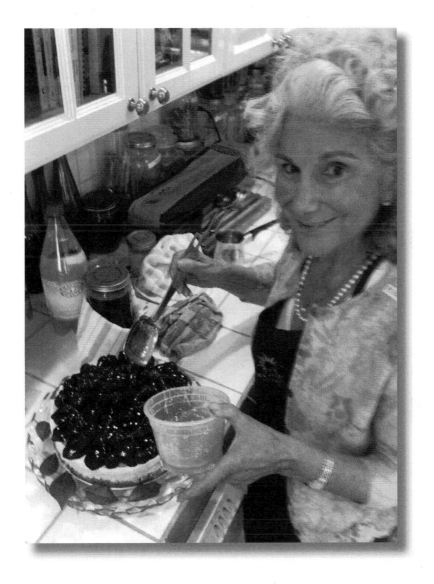

Legendary (from scratch) cheesecake queen.

"Every day of our lives, we are on the verge of making those slight changes that would make all the difference."

–Mignon McLaughlin

Is This the End, Again?

CA 125 (remember that tumor marker?) = all-time high. RAH just called to report from her chemo chair at the cancer center that her number came back higher than when she had full-blown cancer. So, yes, we can say that we are back at that point—full-blown cancer. Shit!

Next steps. *So, just like the first time it was discovered, RAH is attacking it with her oncologist leading the charge. RAH assured the staff today that she will be a great patient and do whatever is needed. Her symptoms have been showing up this past month with a vengeance. She's had some new symptoms too, like halitosis (because of the tumor activity in the liver), along with her reoccurring exhaustion, weakness, hoarseness of voice, and loss of appetite. (RAH is embarrassed about her bad breath.) Note: RAH was unsteady on her feet this morning, so Nicole insisted she use her cane to help her stay stable. RAH told me tonight, when I brought her cane into her bedroom for her to use if she got up to pee, that Nicole insisted she bring it but that she just carried it around. Smart that she had it! RAH opted to go for the biopsy today. She's not wanting to wait for anything she can act on immediately. She texted me that it was "a piece of cake," so tomorrow she'll start a new chemo regimen that will be pretty aggressive and have all the usual, and perhaps new, side effects.*

RAH asked the doctor in front of Nicole today how long he thought she had left to live. He told her that they had to move quickly or that she'd have weeks to months. The cancer was not waiting around for anybody. So, if we don't do any treatment, RAH won't be around longer than a few weeks to months. The doctor told us we'd be seeing a lot of him.

Dear family and friends, thank you for being here, caring, sharing your prayers, your love, light, energy, and time to help us get through this. Here we go (again) . . .

Despair. Deflated. Demoralized. Hopeless. Let's embrace all of that, here and now, shall we? It was heartbreaking to see these things well up in my mom. I felt it all. I could tell by looking at her face, and being in her presence, that she had to face the inevitable. No more ways to "fix this." And now, the "H" word (hospice), which has so many translations depending on who you talk/listen to. By the way, hospice is not a death sentence, by any means, something I didn't realize before this point in our journey. We learned that it's a time when specialists come in to serve the patient and families/caregivers at a different level. That's it. It doesn't mean "the end" is imminent. So, I think that the meaning we put into that word, let alone the paperwork, interviews, and medications that come with it, is completely individual and on a case-by-case basis. For us, it was a "shoring up" of resources because we had no idea what to expect from that point on.

What we found was that we could partner with our wonderful local hospice in caring for our mom, and she could rest and relax, knowing we were being advised by professionals—experts in death and dying, if you will. Hospice care is a wonderful service when the time comes for a loved one who needs another level of care. Some hospice services even provide grief counseling for a period of time, something that was invaluable to me. Use the tools, remember?

Further Inquiry

What is true for you in this moment of your caregiving journey? What are you discovering? Some encouragement for you as you explore these questions: Don't let the "H" word deter or deflate you. Let it lift you up to a Higher love. It is a connection with those who can Help you navigate through it all. Because, as you know, it's a lot. H is for Hospice. What a gift. I had no idea.

"Yesterday is history, tomorrow a mystery, today is a gift. That's why we call it the present."

–unknown

Strength in the Final Months

The chemo is definitely in play. The doctor wasn't kidding when he predicted extreme fatigue. RAH's body has been achy the last few days, and she's had some extreme weakness in her limbs, which proved to put a damper on her evening. We did a ton of organizing most of the day to help RAH feel relaxed and stop worrying about her house not being in order. RAH is keenly aware that she needs to move her body in between rests. Bottom line, the house is ready for company/helpers!

The strength of this little spitfire of a mama, along with her determination to get through these chemo treatments and fight off the cancer, is nothing short of miraculous. She's "not going anywhere," as she continues to reassure us. She knows how the days after chemo go, and we all now realize that we have to keep an even closer eye on her and get more help until she regains her strength, which usually happens after the first few days of chemo.

Thank you, as always, for checking in with us here. RAH wants you to know that she LOVES reading your messages (and when she is too tired to sit at her desk herself, we read them to her). Keep them coming. She is encouraged by your love and prayers, always! Peace.

There was always "doing" around my mom's house. Being productive was bred into me at a cellular level. So there were times, given the reality we were thrust into—a life-and-death reality—that the "doing" seemed like it was another coping mechanism. I guess it makes sense. I've known so many people for whom this is also true. We "do" for so many reasons, not the least of which is to distract ourselves. I wanted to "be" more with my mom, and I also struggled with hovering, something I had practiced in my adult years almost to an art form. There were times my mom wanted me to do things with her, like go out to eat, go shopping, or some other activity. I used to say stuff like "I'd love to play hooky with you, Mom, but I'm not retired yet. You are," and then I'd feel guilty for saying no.

During the final weeks and days of my mom's life, I chose to be as fully present as possible. I let my mom guide me (as well as my family and our hospice team), so that I could be of service. By that time, in contrast to my previous "freaked out" and "what about me?" perspectives, I was ready and prepared for this being-ness.

I let things flow, and truthfully, I had no choice but to relinquish control and breathe.

There's a tension that was always present between the *doing* and the *being* for me. I'm still working that out in every area of my life. What I've learned since my caregiving days is that caregiving is also for caregivers. Myself included. So, while I have this brief moment in time where I'm able to focus on myself so fully, I'm taking advantage of it—I'm learning all the ways I can stay healthy and able to function optimally. I find myself tapping into my whole self, my inner leader, more and more. I am also studying our nervous systems and dabbling in neuroscience here and there. It's all fascinating, and I never realized there is a wealth of learning at hand. Being exposed to so many facets of what it is to be human is a treat and a delight for me. Thankfully, my coach, Tina Meyers, helps me with these things. I think it's important to engage with professionals in our lives who can help us see what we are too close to see by ourselves.

Further Inquiry

When you find the strength you weren't sure you had, where was it? How did you tap into it?

"When you lose a loved one, you suffer. But if you know how to look deeply, you have a chance to realize that his or her nature is truly the nature of no-birth, no-death. Pay attention to the world around you, to the leaves and the flowers, to the birds [and the butterflies] and the rain. If you can look deeply, you will recognize your beloved manifesting again and again in many forms. You will release your fear and pain and again embrace the joy of life."

–Thích Nhât Hanh, *No Death, No Fear*

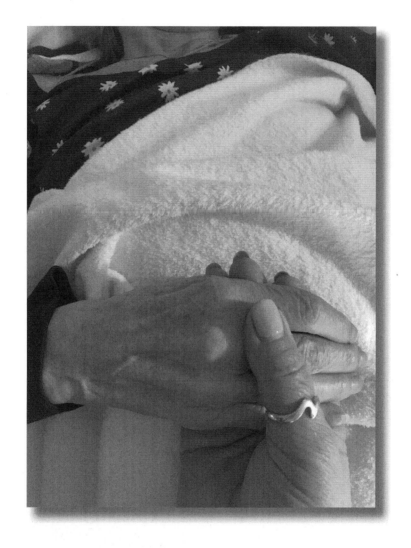

Aware that the final breath is imminent—and she's still "holding me."

LYNN ABATÉ-JOHNSON

Celebrations

RAH was shocked and excited when she arrived at her surprise eightieth birthday party. We held it after an early morning event at her grandson's Senior Speech, which was also a surprise for her in that he spoke about all the lessons his RahRah has taught him throughout his eighteen years so far. We had a crowd of more than fifteen people at the high school gymnasium.

My mom also enjoyed the entire evening even though she was feeling terrible. She perked up, though, being the extrovert she is. Family from Michigan sent video greetings, plus we showed lots of photos and videos of RAH with family and friends over the years. We had a small(ish) intimate gathering of friends and family. People stood up and spoke about RAH and their memories with her. She was flying high, and even the following day, she remarked to me that she felt better than she had in a long time. I said, "Well, Mom, I think you are probably high on love." She agreed.

One of the things that has always bothered me about the way Western culture approaches death is that we have the ritual of a funeral, a memorial, and a celebration of life *after* our loved ones leave us. I think it's completely backward. For this, and many other reasons, I was beyond happy that we were able to shower my mom with all the love, sweet words, beautiful memories, and sentiments that gave her the energy and uplift she felt from that whole day celebration of her life. It not only energized her, but it also let her know how cherished she was while she was alive to enjoy it all. I'm a big proponent of demonstrating every tangible show of love, affection, and gratitude for all people *before* they die, to every extent possible. This also translates into the ways I try to live each day, as challenging as it can be sometimes (especially given family dynamics and relationships that are in flux). I make it a point to lead with love whenever possible. What is new and different about my approach to daily living and loving today is that I now include myself in the loving care that I extend to others so freely. The way I speak to myself and the way I care for myself in all ways is important. It really does make an impact on the ways in which I'm able to be present for my loved ones.

Further Inquiry

Caring for and celebrating yourself is so important. What are some ways that you take care of and celebrate yourself?

"Don't worry about the world coming to an end today. It is already tomorrow in Australia."

–Charles Schulz

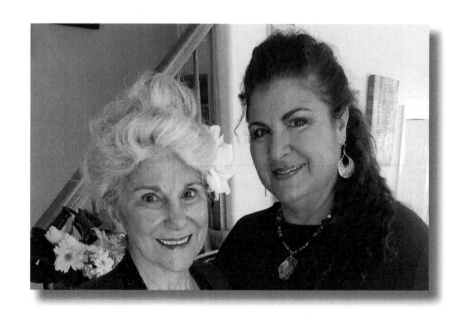

Elegant and excruciating: her 80th birthday.

Love and Respect

The day has come, dear family and friends. RAH, Nicole, and I met with the oncologist and determined that there will be no more chemotherapy administered. The doctor told us that the chemotherapy wasn't tipping the balance in her favor, and that it was time to stop. As the doctor put it (and as we have known for the past five days), RAH has been "running on fumes." Lab work came back with some of the major "players" being way down = not good. And the liver test was also not good. This is a major concern, obviously. The bottom line is that since her last chemo infusion nearly a week ago, RAH has had a very tough time making it through each day without being transported to the ED, so we have gone back to those days when we were on 24/7 watch/care. Nicole stays with RAH every night, and to help with emergencies (as we've had two in the last two mornings) and physical demands, Corey and I are also spending the night to shore up support and serve as extra hands.

Out of love, and my desire to provide a "soft landing" for my beautiful and strong little mama, I grappled with my urge to control the various impacts and outcomes of my mom's physical condition, along with the lab results we were seeing before our eyes. The fact is, however, it was undeniable. We did not have control at that point, at least on physical outcomes. We got advice from hospice, did our own research (as always), and conferred with each other as a family, to do and be whatever was needed in the moments we had remaining together.

Out of respect, we also checked in with each other about personal longings, desires, and preferences. Some of us wanted to be right there with her, while others did not. We included everyone, and nothing was off limits, even after my mom took her last breath. I have no regrets, only love and respect. I think we did a pretty good job overall.

It is so vital in the caregiving journey to draw in the loving humans who love to serve you and your family in some way, shape, or form. I will always remember and be grateful for the loving circle of friends and family members who celebrated alongside us and shored us up from around the globe, out of love!

Further Inquiry

Are there people who have shown up unexpectedly during this time who have been helpers and supporters? I know for me, there were many. Being thankful for the helpers really made a difference during times I felt helpless.

*"Everybody can be great.
Because anybody can serve.
You don't have to have a
college degree to serve.
You don't have to make your
subject and your verb agree to
serve.
You don't have to know the
second theory of thermo-
dynamics in physics to serve.
You only need a heart full of
grace.
A soul generated by love."*

–Martin Luther King Jr.

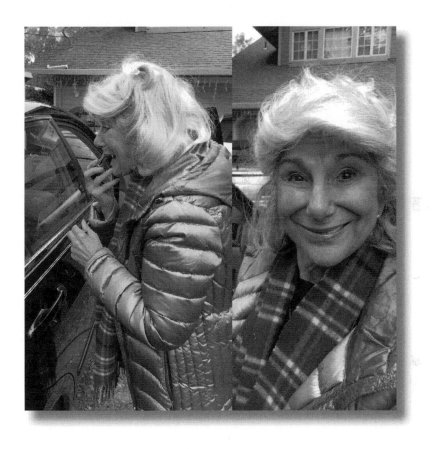

"Mom, remember your lipstick."

Many Hands Make Light Work

All hands on deck. We are revving up for a new phase in care for RAH—tons of scheduling, meetings, research, and development for the plan going forward, which includes support from a new (and amazing!) hospice team, as well as IV VITAMIN infusions. We are also scheduling in dear friends who want to spend time with RAH and look out for her needs (high-impact nutrition, hydration, comfort, exercise, and lots of love).

Thank you so much to those of you who have been helping us care for RAH and to those who are sending cards, gifts, messages. It ALL COUNTS! You ALL matter! RAH is feeling loved and appreciated for all those years of care and love she's been giving to us.

As the end of life approaches, so many emotions and memories flood into the mix. We already had our hands full in navigating new paperwork, new helpers, and new maladies that go with the territory. There was a lot we learned from experience, and there was so much ahead we hadn't yet experienced and had no prior knowledge of. We had to **practice asking for even more help**, by leaning in to friends, family, and strangers who were there to serve my mom as she prepared for her upcoming journey into another realm.

My mom was fiercely independent. She always stepped up to help others figure out their lives by teaching and providing advice and support in every way she could imagine. What she didn't already know, she was determined to learn, but she struggled asking for help because she preferred to be in the role of the helper. She volunteered at her grandchildren's school, cleaning, gardening, making meals for teachers—whatever was needed. Then, when she was diagnosed with ovarian cancer, that same school community stepped up to help support her, her children, and her grandchildren (six of whom were at the school) in many ways, large and small. She learned to accept help and to lean on others as others had always leaned on her.

I know I developed that same sense of independence (often to my own detriment) early in my life. Learning from those years, I have now become more comfortable asking for help and being curious about what is mine to carry, and what is not. We are not meant to carry the weight of the world alone.

Further Inquiry

Where are some places/communities you've been surprised to find kindness and loving support?

"We don't see things as they are, we see things as we are."

–Talmudic idea

Care for the Caregiver

(from somewhere in the middle of the journal entries . . .)
Giving care . . . it's a very special way that we get to serve our little mama. As each hour passes, there is something new and different to observe and adjust with her care. It takes patience and detailed attention, and we communicate (with RAH and between our-selves) through our binder pages, so we don't leave anything to our memories. (Sometimes I think I have chemo brain along with RAH!)

There is always something to do for RAH's care. When she sleeps, we clean up the house, do laundry, keep things fresh around the garden whenever possible, make tea and food for the next small meal, prepare the gear for the upcoming chemo days, work on schedul-ing, gather phone messages and mail, and lots more. When RAH is awake, we hold up the water cup to remind her to sip, offer her bites of food or sips of protein drinks, massage her tummy and feet, prop her up on pillows, help her bathe or shower, clip her nails, find a film for her to watch on TV, and read to her from a book of short stories. There is never a shortage of tasks, even outside the house. It seems we are at the pharmacy a couple times a week, picking up pads and medications for RAH. Inside the home, one of us does the bulk of the grocery shopping, cooks, and someone else organizes/purges the cupboards. Another person brings in the filtered water jugs and keeps the supplements/vitamins well stocked so we can shore up RAH's immune system as much as possible. And then there's all the administrative stuff happening behind the scenes—everything is ongoing.

So, we have an amazing crew of caregivers. It's not for everyone, but the people RAH attracts are extremely focused on her. It's beautiful and heartwarming to see. We couldn't possibly single out caregivers or thank them enough (this is one reason I don't mention a lot of names in my online journal entries).

We consider ourselves so fortunate that RAH has given so much of her love and effort to others and is now receiving gifts (of time and focused energy) from so many to help her rest, heal, and gain nourishment and comfort.

Care for the caregivers. Apparently, this is a "thing" too. Before I was a caregiver, this was an invisible phenomenon to me. In fact, I would have never given myself the label of "caregiver," even though my experience as an empathetic human has thrust me into the role at one time or another.

Being the eldest in my family, I cared for my younger siblings, as well as cousins, and later, friends. If I really peel back layers of my life, I can also see how I put myself into roles of over-responsibility in caring for others, even adults in my life, from a very early age. Being able to care for someone else used to boost my self-confidence (read: ego), even when other parts of my life were shitty (typical adolescence, growing pains, etc.).

It wasn't until I was thrust into being a caregiver for my mom that I thought about that label for myself. And then, just like most things we experience in our lives, all kinds of information, articles, and workshops started coming into my purview. People I already knew and respected or followed on social media were talking about caregiving and caregivers. Yoga for caregivers. Meditation for caregivers. Retreats for caregivers. There's even an amazing profession called "Death Doula" that redefines death and dying in many wonderful and healthy ways. There is a lot of support for caregivers out there, some of which you'll find in the Resources section at the end of this book.

Further Inquiry

What resources can you list for yourself to try, return to, or recommend to others?

"The deeper that sorrow carves into your being, the more joy you can contain."

–Kahlil Gibran, *The Prophet*

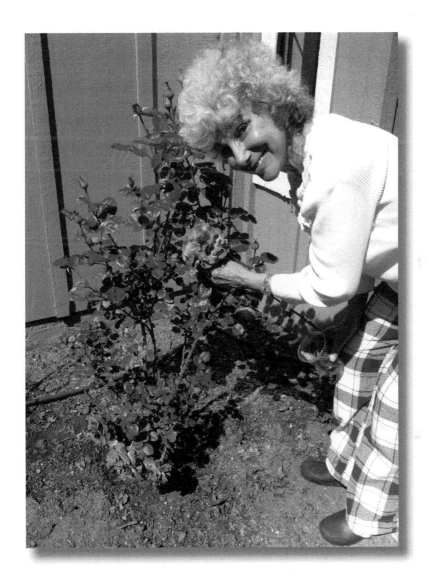

"The Rose Queen"

Coming Clean

We've been living hour by hour this past week as RAH continues on her journey. She is extremely weak most of the time, but she has spurts of energy here and there. Her immune system has taken a beating, obviously, so we have everyone who walks in the house wash their hands first thing. We are also making sure we are feeding RAH as much as we can to boost her system as her organs continue to do their jobs. Most of the time she's still able to walk with us assisting her (we are literally holding her up at times), and she likes having her walker close by so that she feels like if she DOES have the energy, she'll be able to go from the bed to the toilet on her own. When she's too weak to make it to the bathroom on her own, even with the walker, I basically carry her (she's very light and I'm very strong) with the help of a trusty assistant who makes sure her booty lands gently on the "target"/ toilet seat. So this is great, as every visit to the bathroom means that her body is still functioning as it is supposed to. She's been eating and drinking little bits at a time on most days. She has had a couple days that are completely lost to her—she has no recollection of them. There have been times during this period that we haven't been sure whether she'd last through the night.

I can't even imagine going through this journey without my siblings, my husband, and all our kids and dear friends supporting us. Caregiving is not for the faint of heart, and fortunately, RAH has the biggest, strongest heart, so this is all as it was meant to be. Love comes in many forms, and every single bit of it counts.

Coming clean—time to fess up. There was something I'd been skirting around, and after I reread this journal entry, I was reminded that when there are family dynamics and so many unique perspectives in the mix, there may be some fallout in the aftermath of a loved one's death. I'm sad to say that over the years, I've become estranged with some of my family members. When I say I acknowledge all my siblings, I do so with much love in my heart, and also with loving detachment, as I continue to care for myself, learn what's important, and develop and hold personal boundaries. I am responsible to myself and for myself, 100 percent of the time. And so here and now, I am coming clean with the part of my story that has me writing a book without including every individual by name. Every family has its own quirks, personalities, and styles, and I embrace the similarities we share, as well as the differences. It's important to **normalize conflict**, dysfunction, and what I feel as a collective sadness. Since our matriarch has been gone, we have lost that glue that kept us together, exacerbated by differences that always existed. It's assumed by many (in fact, someone said it to me the other day) that I will take over the role of matriarch since I am my mother's firstborn child.

And I used to think that it would be true. I was very wrong. No one becomes the new matriarch, really. No one can fill my mom's shoes in all the ways that she did. Believe me, I tried to be everything to everyone in my family. It didn't work. It doesn't work.

Relationships become what they are meant to become. They are constantly evolving, changing, and morphing. I've found since I've taken a deep dive into my own life that although my family history and relationships certainly inform who I am, they also inspire who I am becoming. And there's another paradox: I have sadness around the loss of my mom and the loss of my living family members in my daily life, while I also have peace and love in my heart as I navigate who I am becoming. Fortunately, I also have the family I choose. I call them Framily—friends who are like family. It's the best feeling to have family members you choose to have, even if you aren't related by blood—those longtime friends who always have your back, regardless of the messiness that transitions and transformations bring.

LYNN ABATÉ-JOHNSON

Further Inquiry

My go-to way of being is four-fold: curiosity, love, gratitude, and acceptance of what is. It is a daily practice for me. On some days, when I start to feel alone, abandoned, or isolated, it is a moment-by-moment practice that helps me stay grounded and not wallow for too long in the dark hole my mind is capable of going to.

What other tools would you add to your toolbox?

"There are two ways of spreading light: to be the candle or the mirror that reflects it."

–Edith Wharton

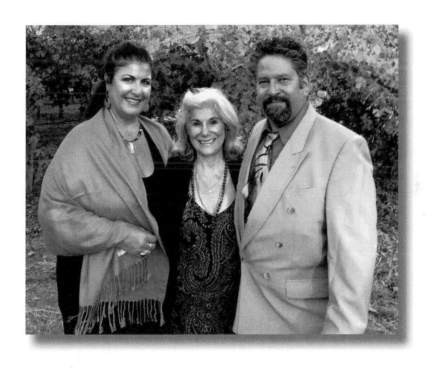

With Corey and me at a wedding.

Journey to the End and the Beginning

Nicole and I started out the day with RAH on a more energetic note (for RAH these days) than yesterday, that's for sure. We have days that I call a "wash," when I am pretty positive my mom does not have a clue what's going on—how many times she's eaten, had something to drink, used the bathroom, gotten her clothes or bedding changed, or any other everyday stuff in the world of our cancer journey. Yesterday was such a day. More and more, it seems like our days are like that, yet underneath all the surface stuff (bodily functions), I keep getting the sense there is some deep internal work happening. My mom is laying groundwork, as she always does. Whether she's in a "state of grace" or "winding down," her mind seems to be fading in and out of the present moment. And yet there is work being done on the inside. We have no way of knowing how many days she has left. It's not up to us, so we are doing our best to keep up with the basics so that she is peaceful and calm and without pain.

So, what makes this journey different today? I considered it a win today when I mixed up a "meal" of five teaspoons of yogurt with supplements blended in. She ate two teaspoons, then waved me off, so I set it aside and waited a while. I let her rest and then went back with the food, which she finished.

I also contemplated the following:

Patience

It's no secret. I was not gifted with natural-born patience. Cancer taught me to step back and breathe. Respect the process for each person individually.

Gratitude

How can we be grateful for a dis-ease that's taking our precious mama/RahRah? We use the tools she taught us. It's one of the best ways to honor and respect her, now and always. I have been finding moments of comfort and joy here and there, with each moment we have left. A few days ago, for instance, we called a family meeting, and all five of us gathered around RAH on her bed. We let her know how much we love her, and each other, that we are all okay, and that she will live on forever in our hearts. We let her know that it's okay to let go. She perked up for a minute and said, "Why are you telling me all these confessions? Where do you think I'm going?" We all cracked up!

Stamina

Just when you think you can't do another thing, you find strength through tenacity, determination, and persistence, and you bounce back. RAH has taught us to be fierce in all we do. It's where each of us gets our special brand of natural intensity. I've learned to embrace that intensity and to use it to get things done, follow through, and be efficient.

Love

Many of you, our friends and family, have called, messaged, written comments here and on our Facebook walls. One of the biggest gifts we have received through all these years is you. The beauty of watching you all love on our precious little mama has been valuable beyond measure. It's like watching RAH when she has us all around, especially her grandchildren. She lights up with delight. Right now, she's not able to light up on the outside, but I can tell when they walk in to say hello and give her a kiss and hold her hand for a moment that she is at peace and happy.

Miracles

We've been beneficiaries of many miracles over the years. RAH has outlived the odds for the advanced dis-ease she started out with in 2011. Is another miracle in store for us? We are definitely open to that, and no one would dare vote against this amazingly strong-willed woman, our mama, our superhero.

Grief

I've always had an interest in watching people. In these past six years, I've tried to step back out of my very involved, personal circumstances around RAH and watch how my immediate family members are doing, starting with my mom, my husband, my siblings, and my nieces and nephews. In the past few months, as we realized we were in for another shit storm (sometimes literally), I've noticed how my mom has embraced the reality of it all, and I've been lucky to be able to have her lead to follow. As I interact with my siblings and their kids, I can see so many ways each is starting to grieve, as RAH is already somewhat gone in the sense that she is so deep inside herself. We can tell her mind is working, but she cannot get the words out in a cohesive sentence most of the time. This is especially affecting the kids, because six years ago, when they were that much younger, they weren't exposed to the worst of RAH's decline. And now, they see it.

When our superhero started to fade, and our roles reversed, we each internalized and interpreted our feelings in unique ways, both for ourselves as individuals and as a family unit.

All the aforementioned characteristics of being human—all the emotions, fears, and joyful moments—are part of this process. Everything is included. Everything is "normal." And as the cliché says, it's okay to NOT be okay at any given moment.

During this time, I was practicing anticipatory grief. I chose this perspective even before my mom took her final breath, without realizing it at the time. And one of my most important values (which became a guiding mantra for me over all the years) is "no regrets."

There's a sort of sweet resignation that I experienced at this stage of the roller-coaster ride. I felt like I was ready to get off the roller coaster, something I've learned is completely normal. How could it not be? With every fiber of being, the caregiver cares about that person who is nearing the end of their life. And the caregiver has been a part of it, all the ups and downs. Those feelings of wanting it to be over need to be normalized, for the caregiver and their loved one. Everyone's ride is the same, and yet each is so very unique.

It helped me to have conversations with myself and others I trusted who were close at hand, to verbalize every single feeling and emotion I was experiencing. I believe it helped me, and helps me to this day, to be okay with missing my mom the way I do. It has normalized the fact that she's gone. It has normalized my loneliness and feelings of abandonment when they surface (and yes, they still do). I use my voice and express exactly what is mine, and mine alone, to express. I seek solace in the experience of others. I know now that it's okay to be vulnerable and ask the questions, while also expressing my longings and desires.

Further Inquiry

As you navigate new territory, what have you discovered about your relationship with the term "normal"? How do you reconcile this within your own heart?

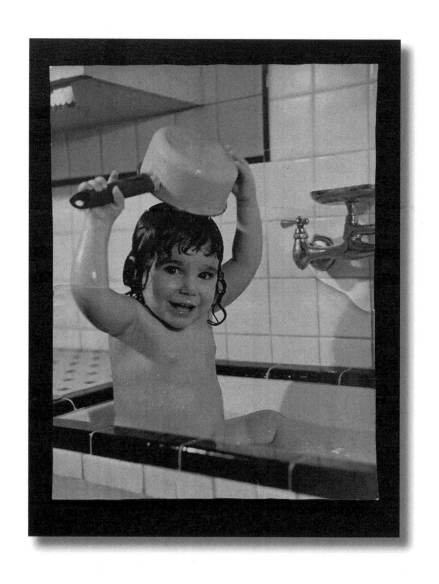

My mom as a baby.

"I want to be thoroughly used up when I die, for the harder I work, the more I live. I rejoice in life for its own sake; life is no brief candle to me. It is sort of a splendid torch which I have got hold of for the moment; and I want to make it burn as brightly as possible before handing it on to future generations."

–George Bernard Shaw

Birthing Stories and Death Stories

The time has come to say "see you later" to RAH.

She has made her transition, peacefully and beautifully.

RAH took her final breath here in Sonoma, California, at 8 a.m., five weeks to the day after her eightieth birthday party.

May 1, May Day, is a day we will always celebrate.

There are spring flowers blooming. RAH passed with her eyes and mouth open, of course. Never one to miss a beat, she guides us, even as she transitioned, finally, to her next adventure. She is with her parents, dear friends, and other family members who preceded her.

To say that we are overflowing with love and appreciation for each and every one of you would be a gross understatement. We are also especially grateful that RAH's wishes were followed to the letter, with no artificial hookups, no morphine or other narcotics

LYNN ABATÉ-JOHNSON

to constipate her, and no hospital bed having to come into the house (she is in her own comfy bed, where she loved being—with the high thread count). We couldn't have asked for more than this.

Before I experienced this journey with my mom, I had so many beliefs and preconceived notions about cancer, dis-ease, death, and dying. I thought things like: death is gross, dying people are gross, funerals are awkward, death is to be feared. I also thought that I wouldn't be able to function without my mom, that losing her would kill me. Yet, I was so wrong on so many levels.

I always loved hearing my mom (and other moms in my life) tell their birthing stories. It's a very wonderful, positive experience and ritual, and these stories are often shared in circles of mothers. Each story is unique, but with many threads of similar aspects as well. It's a joyful occasion for most of us to hear about moms giving birth, adopting, and all the other ways children enter our lives.

I believe much of the same can be said about death stories. (I'm sure there are other terms for it that are more elegant. Or are there? It doesn't matter what we call them.) I believe in the power of our spirits and souls to share our stories with each other as we move through the circle of life (including death). I have come to believe that there is no point in making comparisons; in fact, I think it can be detrimental for all involved. What I know for sure is that we need each other, and the communities we are part of, to create legacies and common truths about being human. When we share our stories about birth and death, we create circles of compassion, love, and understanding. We create healthy perspectives that we can swap with each other, especially when life gets challenging.

Since my intimate experiences with my mom over all those years, and in the aftermath, I now believe our culture has it all wrong about death and dying. I've learned, thanks to my teachers, that there is such a thing as "positive death." As I stated earlier, there's even a profession now called "Death Doula." Until I organically and naturally became a sort of "death doula" with my ride-or-die partner, my wise sister Nicole, I had no clue. I was operating under so many false ideas, and I'm grateful for the experience that led me to view the cycle of life in a way I will no longer shun or avoid.

I have opened my heart, mind, body, and soul to the possibility that death can be positive in many ways. I'm learning so much as I explore what else is possible in our everyday human experience. I wish every caregiver peace, endless curiosity, deep presence through listening (to themselves, their own heart, and to the hearts of others who may guide them), and love.

Further Inquiry

What is your birth story and what is a loved one's death story? Write it all down. What a beautiful gift to give your family and friends during and after life here on earth.

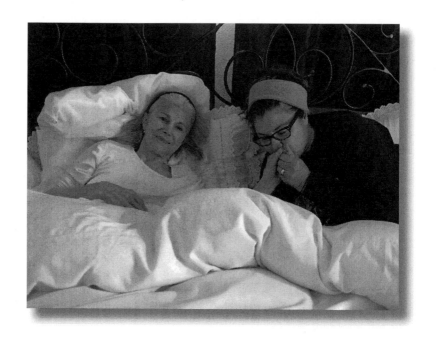

Knowing the end is near in that big fluffy cloud/bed.

LYNN ABATÉ-JOHNSON

"Only when you drink from the river of silence shall you indeed sing. And when you have reached the mountain-top, then you shall begin to climb. And when the earth shall claim your limbs, then shall you truly dance."

–Kahlil Gibran, *The Prophet*

When Does Your Passport Expire?

Surreal. That pretty much sums up this week. Even before RAH took her final breath, I remember being with her and doing normal things like sitting with her for a meal, being in the car going somewhere, or attending an event and having the surreal feeling that one day, this icon in our lives, who I have described as my personal superhero, would be gone from this particular space. So now, her soul is soaring, and we feel her all around us. She's in the flowers outside her kitchen window, in the stars and the sunshine, in her patio fountain, in her big king-sized bed, and especially in all the handwritten notes EVERYWHERE. And the labels. The little silver return-address labels that she plastered on everything. Every pair of scissors, spatula in the kitchen, notepad. And the notes. We are finding it's not so difficult to sort through her things because everything is cataloged and noted. Thus, we have very little guesswork. Thanks, Mom!

*RAH made her feelings and desires very clear to us,
her five "chickens," as she affectionately called us. The
only thing she did not share with us along her journey
was any worry, fear, or trepidation. She never let on,
although we know from our friends who helped us
care for her, that she was only concerned for us. My
theory is that this is the reason she fought so hard
to beat the cancer. She wasn't ready to leave. She
told her best friend, when she was at the end of the
chemo treatments, "I can't believe I'm not going to
beat this thing." With us, she was stoic, humorous,
and unflinching, and she never complained. She was
no victim. She stood strong in the face of all odds
back in 2011, and it took four recurrences for her
to finally leave the body that was no longer serving
her. Right up until her final twenty-four hours, she
knew each of us, including those friends and caregivers who helped us care for her through to the next
adventure. Her surgeon's assistant said in reply to
my email announcement: "What a beautiful way for
her soul to take flight." So true. We are filled with
gratitude for the way that RAH lived and died on
her own terms. Thus far, we smile through our tears
when they hit us in the usual waves of grief. I know
this will continue for some time, and especially once
we are done with the* busyness *of settling her estate.*

As I said, everything is clearly spelled out and written down. She is STILL taking care of us, making sure our processes and systems are efficient. What makes it all a little easier? There are five of us. Those of us who live locally are at her house every single day. Even when we are not doing the work of sorting, organizing, and packing things up, we are here working on our respective jobs. Yes, it's sad that my mom will miss graduations, weddings, and other milestones of life. Still, we are fully able to see the silver linings so far. RAH is able to enjoy each milestone now, free of the dis-ease that eventually took her life.

It's been exactly one week. The grief will be processed differently for each of us, as we are all unique individuals. I think that RAH packed so much living into her life here on earth, and especially the past six years through the cancer journey, that it's pretty difficult to feel sorry for ourselves. Plus, we know that she is still with us in SO many ways.

So, here's something else in the category of "surreal" (and there are plenty of examples): I was collecting RAH's sensitive data/information, and I found all her passports. What fun to look back through those passport photos! Guess what? Her most recent passport expired May 1, 2017 . . . the day she died! Go figure. Always perfect timing, and with style—that's our RAH.

What a freaky thing to discover, isn't it? Someone asked me recently about my experience during the period after my mom's death. They wanted to know what it was like since the daily caregiving ended. What came next? I think this is a worthy exploration. The care doesn't end. It morphs into a different form of care. In my case, I needed to morph into being a caregiver for myself. In fact, I needed to continue learning how to "mother" myself in all the ways in which I had counted on my own mother.

There were also practical aspects of my mom leaving the planet, like her stuff, for example: paperwork, records, files, property (home), and did I mention her stuff? As my mom's administrator (not her executrix), I had the responsibility of managing her papers, files, bills, and all the logistics. I met with the funeral home to arrange for her cremation and to order death certificates, which I did in advance so my mom could weigh in with her opinions. I know this brought some peace of mind for her and also for the rest of us dealing with the emotional aftermath of her death.

Even right up until she started slipping away, my mom noticed the intensity of my facial expressions (usually my crinkled forehead and very stern demeanor). When stressed, I'd make some kind of face, or I'd sigh heavily, and she'd grasp my hand to reassure me: "I'll tell you when to worry."

But she never gave me the "go ahead." She never once said, "Start worrying now because I'm going to die soon, and you'll be without your trusty, strong, forever-young mama." The most reassuring words I've ever heard in my life, however, came from my mom. To this day, I've made a practice of conjuring up her voice in my head, especially when I'm feeling alone, abandoned, rejected, or neglected. "Don't worry, honey," she'd say. "It will all be okay."

When I first heard her diagnosis, through all the fog of swirling thoughts and concern, I felt my world come crashing down around me. Who was going to love me like she did? Who was going to reassure me like she did? Who was going to cook and feed me (while also telling me to lose weight)? Only my mom, Rosemary Ann Hakim. It doesn't matter what my chronological age was, my mom was always the touchstone of my life.

I remember during that first year, when everything was all about me and how I was going to adjust to life on the planet without her, I expressed some of these questions and fears to a friend who told me that I was going to have to learn to be my own mother. How the hell was I supposed to take that on, along with all my other roles, while I was also taking care of others? I struggled with this suggestion for a long while.

Everything was okay, though, just not in the way I wanted it to be. I created a mantra for myself as a way of letting go of control with love. I'd say that my mom was going to "live and die on her own terms" no matter what I did or didn't do. And she did just that.

Further Inquiry
I still imagine my mom's voice in my head: "It's all going to be okay, honey." It amazes me how soothing it is. What words from your loved one(s) are reassuring for you?

"When I sit with my grief, she says, 'You don't have to be afraid of me. I won't swallow you whole. When you feel me, all the way through, I'll bring you back to yourself.'"

–@HillaryLMcBride, Twitter

LYNN ABATÉ-JOHNSON

Mission Critical—Help Others (Be of Service)

I traveled back to Michigan the summer of 2017 for my mom's memorial, which was beautifully planned and executed by some of her siblings there (this is also the place of my birth). I was asked to say a few words, and it felt great to share slices of our lives that we could all relate to, including RAH's fierce determination to have everyone in her family get tested for the BRCA2 gene that caused her cancer. "Knowledge is power," she'd always say. I spoke about RAH's love for children and all the advice she would give to her friends and family about child-rearing over the years, RAH's challenges and persistence as a young wife and mother who moved to California when I was a baby, her intelligence and thirst for knowledge right up until her final week, the way she encouraged us all to manage our finances (by calling to say "turn on the Nightly Business Report!"), and her assurance that her five children made her life worth living, as did her grandchildren and her giant extended Chaldean family and friends. I really enjoyed that day. It was wonderful being joined by so many loving people who showed up to celebrate my mom. There are specific milestones (like birthdays, holidays, anniversaries) to celebrate as we grieve the departure of a loved one, and there are also plenty of other opportunities, if we seek them out, to gather and remember special moments and fun stories. We welcome each and every chance to remember our RAH.

I still love talking about my mom, obviously, since I've woven her into my transformational journey here in these pages. Even in her most intense and traumatic moments, **my mom lived (and died) to serve others**. She was always thinking of people. Aside from all the generous and loving qualities I mentioned at her Michigan memorial service, she enrolled in a study called the Women's Health Initiative. More than 160,000 post-menopausal women ages 50 to 79 participated in the 15-year study, making it one of the largest prevention studies involving women in the United States. She also opted into a Chemotherapy Clinical Trial in 2011 (which nearly killed her). Anytime my mom could help by offering herself as a "test case," she was caring and adventurous enough to do it (once she did her research). Her service to others was a cornerstone of who she was as a human being, a mom, grandmother, sister, aunt, cousin, and friend. A quote by Jack London was framed and displayed in my mom's home. She referred to it enough that we understood the sentiment was important to her, and through her service to others, we watched her demonstrate it.

Further Inquiry

What is your purpose? What are your values, and how are these informing your personal journey as a caregiver?

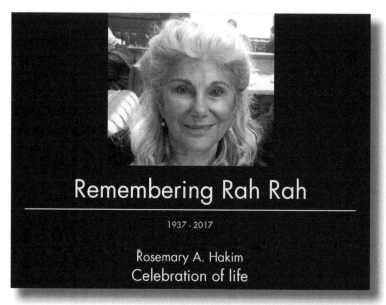

Remembering Rah Rah

1937 - 2017

Rosemary A. Hakim
Celebration of life

For her memorial services.

"I would rather be ashes than dust!
I would rather
that my spark should burn out in a brilliant
blaze than it should be stifled by dry rot.
I would rather be a superb meteor,
every atom of me in magnificent glow,
than a sleepy and permanent planet.
The function of man is to live, not to exist.
I shall not waste my days trying to prolong
them.
I shall use my time."

–Jack London

What's with the Hummingbirds?

Shortly after my mom died, I was having lunch with a good friend, someone who had stepped up to help us care for her. We sat outdoors at the restaurant, and I began noticing hummingbirds everywhere. I had never been surrounded by hummingbirds before, or perhaps I simply hadn't noticed it prior to this day. From May of 2017 on, the hummingbird became "my mom," or at least a symbol of her.

I used to think that hummingbirds never rested, never stopped moving. And that was my mom! She never stopped moving. And yet, in the years since my mom's death, I've seen hummingbirds stop and perch right in front of me, being totally still. I've chosen to interpret this stillness as a metaphor for my new way of being. While I used to flit around being busy, I now have moments when I pause. I no longer feel like I have to be "flapping my wings" during all my waking hours. It has been a revelation, and not an easy thing to do. However, it's been a great practice of mine to lighten up and rest. My newest mantra, one that I never considered before losing my mom, is that "it's not mine to carry."

It seems very simple. Yet in all the years before, when I carried the weight of the world on my shoulders, it manifested in my body. Thus, the layers of fat I packed on for "protection." I don't need it any longer now. I am learning how to be still, to pause, and to express and hold my personal boundaries so that I rarely get hooked or sucked into other people's emotional or physical well-being. If I could learn this lesson from my mom, then perhaps the journey was worth it. She's at peace and no longer fighting, and I am at peace, no longer carrying the excess weight around that was making me sick, tired, and depleted: "the weight of the world!"

Discussions about the aftermath of a loved one's death are so nuanced and layered. There's *doing*, and then as the physical "things" are dispersed and fade away into everyday life, there is *being*. I never used to take the time to *be* with myself. But I'm learning. I have all those existential questions about who I am and where I fit into the world, and I no longer have my mom to discuss them with or to advise me about a choice I need to make. So I'm learning to rely on myself.

I like to joke with my sister Nicole because she is practically a clone of our mom. I relish our time together because it makes me happy that she reminds me so much of her, in ways big and small. It's such a comfort. I also like seeing my mom's things in my siblings' homes. They, like hummingbirds, are wonderful reminders of her.

I feel fortunate that I chose to begin grieving before my mom actually died. There were a couple of nonnegotiables for me during the cancer years: one was to have no regrets, and the other, out of my "realistic optimism," was that I would face the fact that my mom was leaving us after all her years of fighting to live. Her will was there, but her body finally said enough is enough.

Today, these are my lessons, and it is important learning (and UNlearning) for me to continue as I evolve in my leadership journey, as a human being, and as a daughter, wife, sister, aunty, friend, and colleague. **I speak more than ever before about normalizing all the feelings, thoughts, emotions, and challenges that my mom's health journey presented to me.** Being able to look back at all the years on that roller coaster has given me a perspective that is invaluable. There is so much paradox at play. While I miss my mom every day, I don't miss her cancer. (I know that was a part of who she was for a while, but it never defined her.) I've spoken with other daughters/caregivers of moms who have died, and it's reassuring to know that the guilt and relief are perfectly normal. And I realize that the guilt of feeling relieved that my mom is gone is something that not many people, especially loving daughters, would verbalize, much less admit to themselves.

As I write these words, I feel a sadness that she finally had to go. It's Mother's Day 2022, and I'm looking at a beautiful sunset over the Pacific Ocean. I am keenly aware that my story will continue for as long as I walk the planet. I'll always say hi to my mom when I see a hummingbird, smiling because I know that she has never truly gone. Her legacy is strong, and it will always be enough for me. I love you, Mom.

My wish is that you, too, will begin to embrace the paradox and seek support, through candid and constructive conversations, to accept whatever you are experiencing emotionally at any time. We need it all. Everything is included, and no one gets to be right or wrong. This is *your* individual journey as a human being.

Further Inquiry

I hear stories from friends who have been caregivers about how they had conversations with their loved one in which they discussed ways that they might be given a sign that their loved one is still somehow present. Even though I don't remember having such conversations with my mom, the hummingbirds have symbolism for me, which is why when I see them now, I say, "Hi Mom!" Have you had discussions with your loved one(s) related to the time after their departure?

"If you want to bloom, water yourself."

-@PersianPoet, Instagram

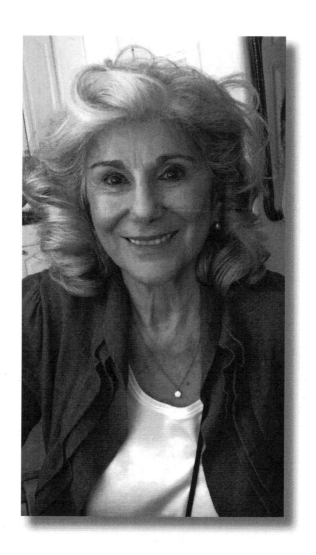

"Hi, Mom" when the hummingbirds visit.

LYNN ABATÉ-JOHNSON

Health after Death

My story as a daughter, caregiver, and human being:

> I needed a moment, a real pause, to say "hello" to me.
> I needed to have some isolation from the system I was immersed in to start getting to know myself.
> I needed time for healing.
> I needed to learn to "mother" myself, with unconditional love.
> I needed to make peace with my body and my hanging/sagging skin.
> I needed to become familiar with my bones, like really feel my own bones and be okay with them.

As I write these words of discovery and transformation, I realize that one of the goals I'm working on is being healthier than I've ever been in my adult life and adjusting to carrying less weight, literally and figuratively. With my loving community of support, I know I'll get there—to self-acceptance and wholeness. It would be so easy for me to wallow and ruminate: *Why couldn't I have figured this out while my mom was still alive so I could have been more of a help to her?* All the "I wishes" flood me sometimes: *I wish she could see me now (she can). I wish she could celebrate with me at this moment (she is). I wish I knew then what I know now (it took her leaving for me to get a clearer perspective).* I am learning to look back on the mistakes I made, especially in regard to my own self-care as a caregiver, and cut myself some slack, as well as extend myself some grace just as I would to anyone else.

In moments of perceived and real crises, there's not much time or space for gentle introspection. I would argue now, however, that if I had realized how much support and services are available for caregivers, I may have been able to tap into my "leader within" much sooner.

I'm here to encourage, inspire, and reassure you. There's support and loving kindness in your circles, and in the wider community. Ask questions, open your heart, and listen to your inner voice that says everything will be okay. It's all so temporary, the struggle and the ease. It's a flow. Each moment has a gift in it, which is often discovered in hindsight. Let this be your assurance that the gifts will find you. Your mission is to allow them in for consideration.

Further Inquiry

What gifts have you uncovered so far in your journey as a caregiver and human being? Be sure to write them down as they come.

"When you are triggered, accept your nervous system reaction unconditionally. This is a time for compassion, finding ease, doing less and supporting yourself. When you are triggered, your survival biology takes over. You have less control over how you react. Make peace with this. Don't blame yourself or try to fix your biology. Ride the waves."

–@AwakenWithAlly, Instagram

Conclusion

Years later, I'm visiting my former hometown, staying at my sister Nicole's. While at the local grocery store where my mom used to shop, I feel a longing for her. I look around, thinking maybe I'll run into her here like I used to. I reminisce about the times I took her shopping when she was too weak to go by herself (when she was feeling well, we could barely keep up with her!). We'd put her in a scooter—disaster! These memories always make me smile and chuckle to myself. Seeing my little mama crashing into store displays . . . what a picture in my head! Fortunately, no one was ever injured and nothing crashed down or broke.

I walk out of the store and glance over at a lady who looks like my mom. I'm taken aback. Talk about a trigger! In addition to being in the store with memories, now I think I've caught a glimpse of her. I am so sad. I tell Nicole how bittersweet it is to be in our hometown, overcome by memories.

In moments like this one, the tears flow. "Feel it to heal it," I tell myself. Let the tears out. Crying is always a cleansing ritual for me that I can never plan for, and it's one that I don't think ever goes away. And that's okay. Memories are precious, and grief is sweet. Let it flow.

"Grief is love look-ing for a home."

–@susandavid_phd, Instagram

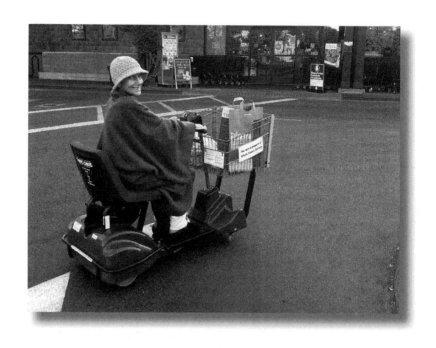

Her driving this cart at the grocery store—funny and scary!

Acknowledgments

I acknowledge my husband, Corey V. Johnson. Not only did he help care for my mom, sit with her when she wasn't feeling well, and watch TV with her, he also cared for our nieces and nephews every time we asked, ran errands, and was 100 percent present with me when we were alone together and I was falling apart. He said to me one time, "Don't apologize for not being at home with me. She's my RahRah too, and I am here for her, and you." And that was the only time he ever needed to say it out loud because he shows up *every single day* and continues to love on me and our extended family as the years have passed. This book would not exist without his support.

I acknowledge my sister, Nicole. Thank you, my bubela, for holding up a mirror for me to see myself through your loving eyes and fierce warrior heart. It is my honor to be your big sister and to have cared for Mom alongside you, every step of the way.

I acknowledge all my siblings. Every one of you stepped up to help care for Mom in the ways you were able to and in the ways you thought best, given none of us had ever experienced this kind of journey.

For my mom, Rosemary Ann Hakim (RAH), who continues to teach me and is a force for empowering transformation in my daily life.

For all the womxn who care deeply and feel profoundly, and especially those who may be neglecting their own health by showing up for their loved ones in such monumental ways.

For all the families who are in the depths of the journey, the "belly of the beast," so to speak. I see you. I feel you. I'm here for you.

For the families grieving the loss of loved ones, and to those who missed the gift of a mom who was present for them in the ways you long for and deserved.

For every family member and friend who walked alongside me in some way or another, as a fellow caregiver, mentor, coach, and so much more—thank you. I will always remember you and your part in this journey, and I wish you well as you navigate your own health journeys.

I acknowledge that I occupy the traditional territory and home-lands of the Luiseño/Payómkawichum people, and I pay respect to their elders, past and present. Luiseño (Loo-sin-yo) Payóm-kawichum (Pie-yom-ko-wi-shum).

And finally, I acknowledge myself. I realize that after all the years have passed, I'm a different person than I was back in 2011 when my mom was diagnosed with ovarian cancer. And ironically, I have transformed my life in the ways my mom would have wanted for me. So hell yes, I acknowledge myself for bringing myself to this point, and I'll continue to become more curious and openhearted in my leadership journey as the years go by.

Resources

Books:

Fouts, Janet. *When Life Hits the Fan: A Mindful Guide to Caring for Yourself While Caring for Others,* Tatu Digital Media, 2018. JanetFouts.com

Gawande, Atul. *Being Mortal: Medicine and What Matters in the End.* Metropolitan Books, 2014. AtulGawande.com

Kessler, David. *Finding Meaning: The Sixth Stage of Grief.* Scribner, 2019.

Perry, Bruce D. and Oprah Winfrey. *What Happened to You? Conversations on Trauma, Resilience, and Healing.* Flatiron Books, 2021.

Petrone, Liz. *The Price of Admission: Embracing a Life of Grief and Joy.* Broadleaf Books, 2020. LizPetrone.com

Speers, Peggi and Tia Walker. *The Inspired Caregiver: Finding Joy While Caring for Those You Love.* CreateSpace, 2013.

van der Kolk, Bessel. *The Body Keeps the Score: Brain, Mind, and Body in the Healing of Trauma.* Penguin, 2015. BesselvanderKolk.com

van der Kolk, Bessel. *Workbook—The Body Keeps the Score: Brain, Mind, and Body in the Healing of Trauma.* 2021.

Zuba, Tom. *Permission to Mourn: A New Way to Do Grief.* Lightning Source, 2014. TomZuba.com

Coaching and Programs:

Rachel Baldi, End-of-Life Coach: RachelBaldi.com

Danielle LaPorte, Creator of The Heart Centered Leadership Program: DanielleLaporte.com/the-goddess-of-grief-getting-to-the-other-side-and-there-is-always-another-side (2021)

Tina Meyers, Intuitive Coach, Creator of Women Advocates Rising and Warrior School: WomenAdvocatesRising.com

Grief and End of Life Training, Coaching, and Advocacy at UpLevel Productions: UplevelProductions.com.

Co-Active Training Institute: coactive.com

Additional Support:

Bridget Foliaki-Davis, Chef, Nutritionist, Author: YouTube.com/c/TheInternetChef

California Caregiver Resource Centers: CaregiverCalifornia.org

Caringbridge.org—share online health updates, photos, and videos with the people who care about you and your loved one(s)

Family Caregiver Alliance: Caregiver.org

Teri Portugal Gooden, Certified End-of-Life Doula Professional: Infinite-Passage.com

Miscellaneous:

Administration For Community Living: ACL.gov

National Family Caregiver Support Program [NFCSP], established 2000: ACL.gov/programs/support-caregivers/national-family-caregiver-support-program

National Library of Medicine: NLM.nih.gov

Square Breathing Technique and more: https://blog.zencare.co/square-breathing (2022 Zencare Group, Inc.)

Women's Health Initiative: WHI.org

For additional resources, please visit: LynnAbateJohnsonBook.com

Works Cited

Anagnost-Repke, Angela. https://www.mother.ly/parenting/dear-daughter-be-loud-take-up-space-your-voice-matters/

Angelou, Maya. *I Know Why the Caged Bird Sings*. Random House, 1969.

Brown, Brené. *Daring Greatly: How the Courage to Be Vulnerable Transforms the Way We Live, Love, Parent, and Lead*. Avery, 2012.

Bucchianeri, E.A. *Brushstrokes of a Gadfly (Gadfly Saga)*. Batalha, 2011.

Faulds, Danna. dannafaulds.com

Gibran, Kahlil. *The Prophet*. Alfred A. Knopf, 1973.

Kessler, David. *Finding Meaning: The Sixth Stage of Grief*. Scribner, 2019.

LaPorte, Danielle. DanielleLaporte.com

Nin, Anaïs and Gunther Stuhlmann. *The Diary of Anaïs Nin Volume 5*. Harcourt, 1974.

Raheem, Octavia. *Pause, Rest, Be: Stillness Practices for Courage in Times of Change*. Shambhala, 2022.

Speers, Peggi and Tia Walker. *The Inspired Caregiver: Finding Joy While Caring for Those You Love*. CreateSpace, 2013.

Shaw, George Bernard. *Man and Superman*. 1903.

Thích Nhất Hanh, *No Death, No Fear: Comforting Wisdom for Life*. Riverhead, 2002.

Williamson, Marianne. *A Return to Love: Reflections on the Principles of "A Course in Miracles."* HarperPerennial, 1993.

Biography

Lynn Abaté-Johnson has provided a unique guidepost for living during uncertain, frightening years as an all-of-a-sudden caregiver for her mom, as well as in the years since her mom's death from ovarian cancer. Her words offer a personal glimpse into her journey as a daughter of a strong mother, with a particular focus on her own transformation in the aftermath of being a caregiver.

Lynn's approach helps to remove the stigma of grief and all that accompanies its journey, both before and after the death of her mom. Her expressive and often vulnerable ways of sharing help to normalize what many families may take for granted or miss in their often-overwhelming and new experience as caregivers. There will be discomfort, shame, guilt, and layers of conditioning to discover in this book, with the goal of bringing light to the dark and peace to the soul.

This book is also interactive: you will find practical, logistical resources on the accompanying website: LynnAbateJohnsonBook.com.

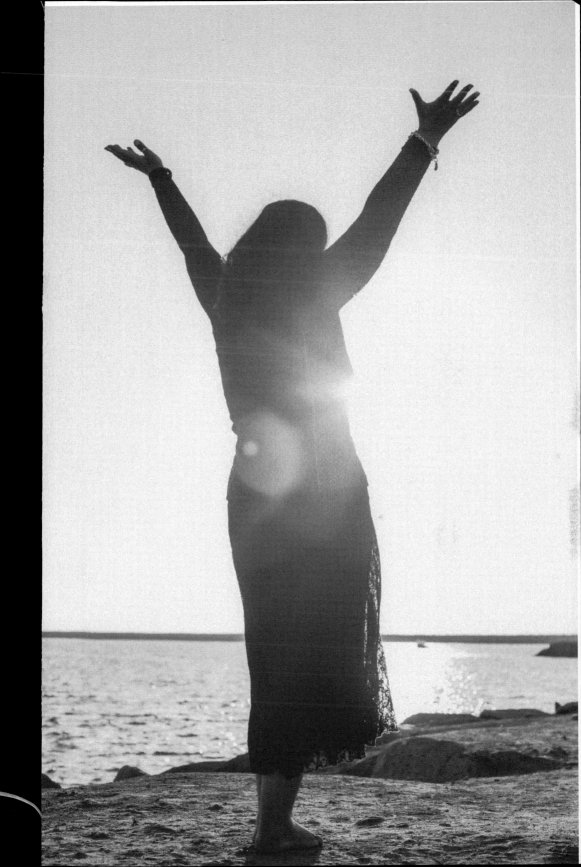